DEDICATION

To my mother, Ruth, who always makes everything comforting.

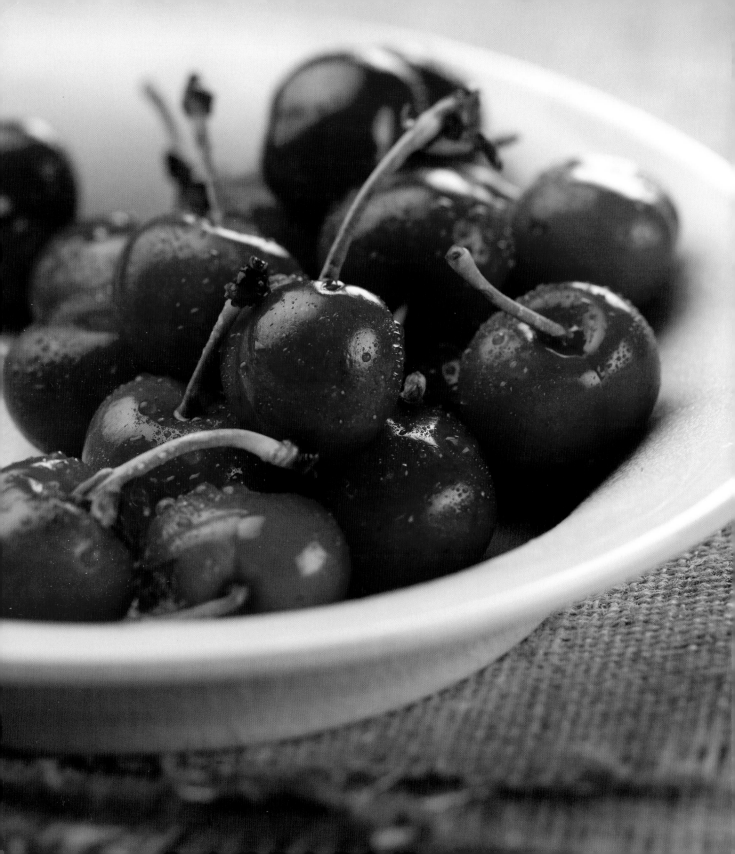

Table of Contents

Acknowledgments | vi

Introduction | vii

CHAPTER 1 Comfort Food Starters | 1

CHAPTER 2 Sides and Salads | 17

CHAPTER 3 Soups and Stews | 43

CHAPTER 4 American Classics | 63

CHAPTER 5 International | 93

CHAPTER 6 One Pot and Skillet | 111

CHAPTER 7 Pasta | 127

CHAPTER 8 Desserts | 143

APPENDIX Selecting and Storing Vegetables | 171

Index | 175

Acknowledgments

Comfort food usually evokes images of many gathered around the table. Here are my "many" who gathered around my table and who made this book come to be.

First, I'd like to extend many thanks to Abe Ogden, Director of Book Publishing, for making sure this book happened. I thank him for his wisdom, support, and encouragement throughout my many long years as an author and food editor for the American Diabetes Association, and to Rebekah Renshaw, developmental editor, for her guidance overseeing and coordinating every piece of this project.

Thanks go to the fabulous team of Renee Comet, Lisa Cherkasky, Carolyn Schimley, Matt Batista, and Marguerite Bottorff, who beautifully created my food in pictures. Their meticulous commitment to detail and perfection is a rare quality and I am so grateful to have their tremendous talent on my team.

Thanks to pixiedesign, llc, for the beautiful design and typesetting of the book. It really captures the essence of Comfort Food.

Always, thanks are extended to my agent, Beth Shepard, who has stood by me through many many years of creating interesting projects. Her insight and foresight into what showcases my talents best is what every cookbook author dreams about; I'm grateful for her guidance every day.

Gathering around my table is the best team of recipe testers and developers I have ever had for a cookbook project. These fine people tested and retested until a recipe was perfect. All of them made the right judgments when it came to tweaking a recipe, so they are all more than just testers, they should be credited as recipe developers as well. Many thanks go to Anna Berman, Olga Berman, Pam Braun, Arianna Delorenzi, Donna Douglass, Ramzi Faris, Derek Lee, Amanda Markulec, Scott Naples, Kathy Pandol, Kristina Razon, and Cecilia Stoute. They worked tirelessly to make sure every recipe tastes delicious.

I love having colleagues who share my enthusiasm for great tasting food. They generously contributed fabulous comfort foods to my book and I am ever indebted. Andy Bellatti, RD, Corinne Dobbas, RD, Aviva Goldfarb, Molly Morgan, RD, Janel Ovrut, RD, Alexandra Oppenheimer, Robin White, and Elisa Zied, RD, your recipes have made my comfort food book that much more scrumptious.

And finally to all my readers who have stuck by me for so many years knowing that food for people with diabetes means fabulous food at every meal.

Introduction

Many years ago, I made a commitment to travel around the world as much as I possibly could. Of course I was interested in the history and culture of the countries that I visited, but mostly I wanted to learn about the social aspects of each culture; particularly how food plays an integral part of daily life from everyday meals to holiday feasting and celebrations. I've also had the opportunity to dine at some the world's foremost restaurants and sample intriguing and exotic dishes. But when I think of my fondest food memories, I realize my favorite dishes are the simple ones prepared in quaint establishments where I was able to chat with the cook behind the stove. It was the comfort foods of each country: a rustic stew, pasta simply dressed with freshly pressed olive oil and garlic, and perfectly roasted potatoes that I swear I can still taste when I conjure up memories of my travels.

Comfort foods are truly the foods that bind us together. They have stories to tell and the ability to make everything seem just a little bit better on a cold and rainy day. But most of all, comfort foods are the foundation of great cooking. It was actually my mom's perfect meatloaf, her crisp roast chicken, and even her paprikash straight from her Hungarian heritage that taught me the fundamentals of cooking. My mom, by the way, has had diabetes for the past 48 years and if she has learned to manage it by preparing comfort foods, it was time for me to write this book.

When you think of comfort foods, typically rich, fattening, and forbidden foods come to mind. When people are first diagnosed with diabetes, they fear that all of the foods they cherish will be eliminated in favor of sparse, bland food. Recognizing this, I saw the need for a cookbook filled with familiar foods that would meet the dietary needs of those with diabetes. The fact is I have had more success with my own nutrition clients when I tell them they can have their favorite comfort foods and all they need to do is tweak the kind of fat, and the quantity and type of sugar and sodium. And that's what *The Diabetes Comfort Food Cookbook* is all about. Here you'll find *Mac 'N' Cheese*, *Meatloaf*, *Chicken Pot Pie*, *Mashed Potatoes*, *Turkey Stroganoff*, *Brownies*, and even a *Fudge Pudding Cake*. The book is divided into Starters, Sides and Salads, Soups and Stews, American Classics, International, One Pot and Skillet, Pasta, and of course, Desserts. The recipes in each chapter will hopefully be familiar to you and that's a good thing. All I've done is a little tweak here and there to bring you a dish that is diabetes friendly while remaining true to its comfort food roots.

When you choose a recipe to prepare, first and foremost, choose the very best-quality foods you can find and afford. This does not necessarily mean expensive, it means that you'll need to be more informed about your food choices. Read labels, find out the source of the produce you are buying, and ask for locally grown meats and produce at your grocer. Visit your local farmers market for fresh and seasonal produce and other products. Buy the very best-quality cocoa available (not one laden with sugar or chemicals) and your chocolate desserts will taste better every time.

The cooking methods used in this book are intended to give you maximum flavor. Instead of bland steamed vegetables, you'll find oven-roasted vegetables with heightened sweetness and increased flavor. Lean meats are paired with simple savory sauces so you get great taste in every bite.

And when it comes to fat (a main flavor quotient determining whether food will taste delicious or flat), I don't eliminate fat or use a diet substitute. Real olive oil and real butter are used in small amounts: just enough so all the flavors meld together in a dish. I recommend shopping wisely for good quality oils and try European-style butter. European butter is so rich you need only the tiniest amount to make your recipes sing.

When it comes to using cheese (the cornerstone of comfort food cooking), reducing the quantity of cheese or using reduced-fat cheese is key. Small amounts of reduced-fat cheeses are used and I suggest taste-testing a few brands before you choose one. I also use real Parmesan cheese. Buy a wedge of Parmesan cheese to have on hand, not the canned variety.

While you'll see salt listed as an ingredient in many of the recipes, I recommend using salt "to taste" and that you use kosher or sea salt instead of a plain iodized salt. Kosher or sea salt makes food shine. The way the salt crystals are cut helps to bring out the flavor in foods unlike iodized salt, which often overpowers and masks flavors. Don't forget to use fresh and dried herbs and ground spices; while not substitutes for salt, they give any dish an aromatic and fresh taste.

Sugar is always the subject of debate when it comes to the management of diabetes and I tried to stick as closely as possible to the original versions of favorite desserts. I do use sugar but in combination with another one of my new favorite sweeteners, stevia. Well it's not exactly new, it's been around for over 400 years, but I'm new to using it. Stevia comes from a plant that grows in South America, Malaysia, and other parts of the world. The leaf is sweet and its sweetness is extracted by brewing it (similar to tea). The result is a sweetener that can be used alone or in combination with sugar for baking. It is completely natural, and has no calories or carbohydrates. All recipes in this book that contain stevia were tested using Stevia Extract in the Raw. I also use Splenda. It's a familiar product that still delivers good baking results. Occasionally, I only sweeten a dish with small amounts of honey or sugar. The key to controlling excessive carbohydrates is not exclusive to using sugar substitutes; the key is reducing portion size. I'd rather create satisfying smaller desserts made with real ingredients, than artificially sweetening a huge portion. Besides, it's a great exercise in portion control, which is an added benefit.

Many health professionals believe that one should "eat to live." In many ways this belief is a logical step toward good health. I have a bolder vision of wellness. My belief is that it's actually okay to "live to eat." Eating well is one of life's greatest pleasures. Health to me is more than a great checkup with your doctor or a number on a scale. Good health encompasses an attitude of happiness and pleasure derived from daily activities. If eating can give a joyful experience beyond its nutritional makeup, I believe that you can find balance between what we need to eat for good health and what makes our taste buds dance in delight. It is my hope that this book will fulfill that goal.

To life with great taste, enjoy!

Robyn Webb

Hamburger Sliders with Dijon Mustard Sauce, p. 9

CHAPTER 1

Comfort Food Starters

Asian Chicken Dumplings | 2

Cheddar Baked Potato Skins | 3

Classic Hummus | 4

Crab Louis | 5

Creamy Crab Spread | 6

Creamy Deviled Eggs | 7

Double Cheese Pizza Bites | 8

Hamburger Sliders with Dijon Mustard Sauce | 9

Roasted Chickpeas | 10

Sausage Stuffed Mushrooms | 11

Spanish Style Dates with Bacon | 13

Savory Ginger Beef BBQ Appetizer | 14

Sweet Onion, White Bean, and Artichoke Dip | 15

SERVES 12 SERVING SIZE 2 dumplings PREPARATION TIME 25 minutes COOK TIME 4 minutes per 4–5 dumplings

Asian Chicken Dumplings

3/4 pound lean ground chicken

1/2 cup thinly sliced scallions

1/4 cup peeled, shredded carrot

1/4 cup minced water chestnuts

1/4 cup chopped cilantro

4 teaspoons reduced-sodium soy sauce

1/2 teaspoon ground ginger

pepper, to taste

24 wonton wrappers

SAUCE

6 tablespoons reduced-sodium soy sauce

3 teaspoons rice vinegar

2 teaspoons toasted sesame oil

1 teaspoon toasted sesame seeds

1 teaspoon sugar

1/4 cup sliced scallions

I always include this recipe when I teach children. It's great fun and really gets kids involved. But make no mistake, the flavors in these dumplings are complex and adults love them too.

1 In a medium bowl, combine the chicken, scallions, carrot, water chestnuts, cilantro, soy sauce, ginger, and pepper.

2 Working with several wrappers at a time, fill the wontons. Place a teaspoon of filling on the bottom half of the wonton. With a wet finger or pastry brush, moisten the sides of the wonton. Fold the sides over the filling to form a triangle. Repeat with all wontons. Place all the dumplings on a plate or baking sheet and cover with a towel.

3 Combine all sauce ingredients in a bowl.

4 Fill a large stockpot two-thirds full with water. Heat the water to simmering. Removing the dumplings from under the towel, add the dumplings, about 4–5 at a time, and cook for about 4 minutes as they float to the top. Remove the dumplings with a slotted spoon or skimmer. Place cooked dumplings on a plate and keep warm. Repeat with remaining dumplings, keeping them covered with the towel until they are ready to be placed in the water. Continue to cook each batch of dumplings for about 4 minutes. Drain and serve with sauce.

EXCHANGES/
CHOICES

1/2 Starch
1 Lean Meat

Calories **95**
  Calories from Fat **30**

Total Fat **3.5 g**
  Saturated Fat **0.8 g**
  Trans Fat **0.0 g**
Cholesterol **25 mg**

Sodium **435 mg**
Total Carbohydrate **9 g**
  Dietary Fiber **1 g**
  Sugars **2 g**
Protein **7 g**

2 | The Diabetes Comfort Food Cookbook

Cheddar Baked Potato Skins

4 small (about 4 ounces each) baking potatoes

1/2 cup reduced-fat shredded cheddar cheese

1/2 cup nonfat sour cream

2 scallions, minced

I remember when potato skins were all the rage back in the 1980s. Gooey cheese nestled inside a baked potato shell is so simple, who doesn't clamor to gobble them all up? Add a bit of diced bacon if you wish, but cheese and potatoes are all you need to have a great comfort food appetizer.

1   Preheat the oven to 400°F. Scrub the potatoes well. Pierce each potato with a fork. Bake the potatoes for 45 minutes until tender. Remove from the oven and let cool.

2   When the potatoes have cooled, cut them in half lengthwise. Scoop out and discard the pulp, leaving a 1/2-inch-thick shell. Sprinkle the shells with the cheese.

3   Place the potatoes on a baking sheet and bake at 400°F for about 15 minutes until the cheese is bubbly. Transfer to a serving platter and top each skin with sour cream and scallions.

EXCHANGES/ CHOICES	Calories **65** Calories from Fat **15**	Sodium **80 mg** Total Carbohydrate **10 g**
1/2 Starch 1/2 Fat	Total Fat **1.5 g** Saturated Fat **1.0 g** Trans Fat **0.0 g** Cholesterol **5 mg**	Dietary Fiber **1 g** Sugars **1 g** Protein **3 g**

Classic Hummus

1 15-ounce can chickpeas, drained

3 tablespoons sesame tahini

2 tablespoons olive oil

3–4 garlic cloves, chopped

juice of 1 large lemon

kosher salt, to taste

freshly ground black pepper, to taste

Never purchase store-bought hummus again! I'm always surprised that my cooking students don't know how to make hummus. It's so easy; plus, you can regulate the amount of fat in it. Really, the only issue with store-bought hummus is that it is too high in fat. Making your own solves that problem in a pinch. This is the classic version and, as far as I am concerned, this is the only hummus recipe you will need.

1   In a food processor or blender combine all ingredients until smooth, but thick. Add water if necessary to produce a smooth hummus.

2   Store covered for up to 5 days.

EXCHANGES/ CHOICES

1 Carbohydrate
1 High-Fat Meat

Calories **155**
  Calories from Fat **90**
Total Fat **10 g**
  Saturated Fat **1.3 g**
  Trans Fat **0 g**
Cholesterol **0 mg**

Sodium **85 mg**
Total Carbohydrate **14 g**
  Dietary Fiber **4 g**
  Sugars **2 g**
Protein **5 g**

Off the Shelf Appetizer Ideas

CHEESE AND FRUIT BRUSCHETTA

Cut some French bread into 1/3-inch slices. Brush lightly with olive oil. Toast in the oven until very lightly browned. Top with a small piece of low-fat cheese. Return to oven to melt the cheese under the broiler. Top with a sprinkle of dried cranberries or cherries.

SHRIMP MARTINIS

Thaw frozen large, cooked shrimp. Add shrimp to a martini glass with chopped red onion, some capers, and a dollop of nonfat Greek yogurt. Sprinkle with fresh chopped dill.

VEGGIE PITA TRIANGLES

Brush whole-wheat pita bread with olive oil. Place pita bread on a baking sheet and toast for 2 minutes in a 400°F oven. Remove the pita bread from the oven and top with jarred roasted red pepper strips, sliced olives, and drained water-packed halved artichoke hearts. Cut into triangles and serve.

Crab Louis

DRESSING

1 cup nonfat mayonnaise

3 tablespoons ketchup

2 tablespoons minced scallions

1 tablespoon Worcestershire sauce

1 tablespoon red wine vinegar

1 tablespoon lemon juice

1 teaspoon hot sauce

kosher salt, to taste

freshly ground black pepper, to taste

lettuce leaves

1 pound cooked fresh lump crabmeat

1 medium cucumber sliced

1 large tomato, halved and sliced

There was a time in culinary history when food had regal names. Some of them actually tasted quite good despite the very silly monikers. Crab Louis is one of them. It makes a great comfort food with its creamy dressing and serves as a great beginning to any meal.

1 In a bowl, combine the mayonnaise, ketchup, scallions, Worcestershire sauce, red wine vinegar, lemon juice, hot sauce, salt, and pepper and mix well. Cover and refrigerate for 30 minutes.

2 For each serving, line an appetizer plate with lettuce leaves. Add the crab, drizzle with dressing, and garnish each plate with cucumbers and tomatoes.

EXCHANGES/ CHOICES		
1/2 Carbohydrate 1 Lean Meat	Calories **90** Calories from Fat **15**	Sodium **440 mg** Total Carbohydrate **8 g**
	Total Fat **1.5 g** Saturated Fat **0.3 g** Trans Fat **0.0 g**	Dietary Fiber **1 g** Sugars **5 g**
	Cholesterol **50 mg**	Protein **11 g**

Creamy Crab Spread

1/2 cup minced celery

1/2 cup minced red pepper

1/2 cup reduced-fat cream cheese

1/3 cup nonfat mayonnaise

1 tablespoon minced parsley

1 teaspoon hot sauce

1/2 teaspoon lemon zest

sea salt, to taste

freshly ground black pepper, to taste

1 pound lump crabmeat, picked over to remove any shells

Healthy appetizers shouldn't be just about munching on some dried out carrot sticks and limp celery. Join the party with this creamy crab dip brightened with fresh lemon zest and chunks of ocean-fresh crabmeat.

1 Combine all the ingredients (in the order given) in a bowl. Mix well. Serve with crudités.

EXCHANGES/ CHOICES

1 Lean Meat

Calories **50**
Calories from Fat **20**

Total Fat **2.0 g**
Saturated Fat **1.0 g**
Trans Fat **0.0 g**

Cholesterol **45 mg**

Sodium **155 mg**

Total Carbohydrate **1 g**
Dietary Fiber **0 g**
Sugars **1 g**

Protein **6 g**

Quickie Nonfat Greek Yogurt Dips

Start with 2 cups plain, nonfat Greek yogurt and make one of the following for a delicious dip for cut carrots, zucchini, celery, broccoli, or cauliflower:

DILL DIP

To the Greek yogurt, add 3 tablespoons chopped fresh dill, 1/2 teaspoon fresh lemon juice, 1 minced garlic clove, and 2 tablespoons finely minced onion. Blend well and serve.

VEGGIE DIP

To the Greek yogurt, add 1 small red pepper, minced; 1/2 small minced red onion; 2 garlic cloves, minced; 2 tablespoons minced fresh parsley; and 1 tablespoon minced fresh basil. Blend well and serve.

CURRY DIP

To the Greek yogurt, add 1 tablespoon curry powder, 1 tablespoon lemon juice, and 1/2 teaspoon Worcestershire sauce. Blend well and serve.

Creamy Deviled Eggs

12 large eggs

3/4 cup nonfat sour cream

2 scallions, finely chopped

1/3 cup finely chopped
green bell pepper

1/3 cup finely chopped red
bell pepper

2 teaspoons Dijon mustard

sea salt, to taste

freshly ground black
pepper, to taste

3 tablespoons finely
chopped parsley

paprika, for dusting

Deviled eggs have got to be one of the ultimate comfort foods. True, they are a bit old fashioned, but to me they never go out of style.

1 Bring eggs and cold water to a full boil uncovered in a large saucepan. Remove from heat, cover, and let stand 15 minutes. Rinse eggs under cold water to cool them. Peel eggs, cut lengthwise in half, and remove yolks. Discard 8 yolks.

2 Arrange 20 egg white halves on platter. Chop remaining 4 egg white halves very finely. Mash 4 yolks with fork. Transfer whites and yolks to medium bowl. Stir in sour cream, scallions, green and red peppers, mustard, salt, and pepper.

3 Pipe or spoon egg mixture into egg white halves. Sprinkle with parsley and dust with paprika.

EXCHANGES/ CHOICES	Calories **60** Calories from Fat **20**	Sodium **115 mg** Total Carbohydrate **4 g**
1 Lean Meat 1/2 Fat	Total Fat **2.0 g** Saturated Fat **0.7 g** Trans Fat **0.0 g** Cholesterol **85 mg**	Dietary Fiber **0 g** Sugars **2 g** Protein **6 g**

Double Cheese Pizza Bites*

3 cups all-purpose flour, divided

1 teaspoon sugar

1 packet rapid-rise yeast

1 cup very warm water (120 to 130°F)

1 tablespoon olive oil

salt, to taste

1 pint cherry tomatoes, thinly sliced

2 ounces Fontina cheese, shredded

3 tablespoons freshly grated Parmesan cheese

12 Kalamata olives, pitted and cut into slivers

fresh oregano leaves

Instead of a full slice of carb- and calorie-laden pizza, try these little flavor packed pizza bites. The Fontina cheese adds an intense flavor and cherry tomatoes are delicious all year round.

1   Mix 1 cup flour, sugar, and yeast in bowl. Stir in the water and oil until blended. Pulse 1 3/4 cups flour and salt in food processor to mix. Add yeast mixture and pulse until blended. With motor running, add remaining flour, 1 tablespoon at a time, until soft dough forms, about 30 seconds.

2   Dust work surface lightly with flour. Turn out dough and knead until smooth, 1 to 2 minutes. Shape into ball. Cover with clean kitchen towel and let rest 10 minutes.

3   Preheat oven to 450°F. Line two baking sheets with parchment paper. Divide dough into 4 pieces. Wrap the 4 dough pieces in plastic and place in the refrigerator for 1/2 hour.

4   Remove the 4 dough pieces from the refrigerator and cut each of them into 3 equal pieces (for a total of 12 small rounds of dough); shape each into 1 1/2-inch balls. With a rolling pin, roll out each ball into 3-inch rounds. Arrange on baking sheets. Lightly coat each pizza round with nonstick cooking spray.

5   Top each pizza with 2 or 3 tomato slices. Sprinkle with Fontina and Parmesan cheeses, plus a few olive slivers and oregano leaves. Bake until bubbly and crust is golden, about 10 minutes.

EXCHANGES/ CHOICES		
1 1/2 Starch 1 Fat	Calories **130** Calories from Fat **35**	Sodium **85 mg** Total Carbohydrate **26 g**
	Total Fat **4.0 g** Saturated Fat **1.4 g** Trans Fat **0.0 g**	Dietary Fiber **1 g** Sugars **2 g**
	Cholesterol **5 mg**	Protein **5 g**

*Adapted from *Eat To Beat Diabetes* (Readers Digest, 2007)

Hamburger Sliders with Dijon Mustard Sauce

1 1/2 pounds 93% lean ground beef

2 tablespoons minced parsley

2 tablespoons very finely chopped onion

kosher salt, to taste

freshly ground black pepper, to taste

SAUCE

1/2 cup fat-free mayonnaise

1 tablespoon coarse Dijon mustard

2 teaspoons drained capers

1 teaspoon fresh lemon juice

dash hot sauce

15 whole-wheat cocktail-sized buns or pita breads, split

15 baby arugula leaves

Sliders are all the rage now. Since they are usually on bar food menus, you'd think they were off limits to anyone watching their health. By making them yourself, it's like having your own cocktail hour at home. These are a perfect example of portion control. Turn them into dinner by adding a salad and a side of cooked vegetables.

1 Preheat the oven to 400°F. Line a baking sheet with parchment paper and set aside.

2 In a bowl, mix together the beef, parsley, onion, salt, and pepper. Mix until just combined. Do not over handle the beef. Form into 15 mini burgers and set aside.

3 Combine all the ingredients for the sauce and set aside. Add the split breads to the prepared baking sheet. Toast the breads lightly, about 2–3 minutes.

4 Meanwhile, coat a grill pan with nonstick cooking spray. Heat the grill to medium. Grill the mini burgers about 4–5 minutes per side, turning once.

5 To assemble: place a mini burger on one piece of the bun or pita bread. Top with an arugula leaf. Add a dollop of sauce. Place remaining bun or pita bread half on top.

EXCHANGES/ CHOICES	Calories **105**	Sodium **255 mg**
	Calories from Fat **40**	Total Carbohydrate **16 g**
1 Starch	Total Fat **4.5 g**	Dietary Fiber **2 g**
1 Med-Fat Meat	Saturated Fat **1.5 g**	Sugars **3 g**
	Trans Fat **0.2 g**	Protein **11 g**
	Cholesterol **30 mg**	

Roasted Chickpeas

2 cups chickpeas, drained and rinsed

3 teaspoons olive oil

1/2 teaspoon kosher salt

1/2 teaspoon ground cumin

1/2 teaspoon ground coriander

1/4 teaspoon ground red pepper

1/4 teaspoon ground black pepper

Nuts are a highly nutritious food, but the fat content can get out of hand when you're eating them by the handfuls, as many people do. Here's another way to serve a crunchy snack that's far lower in fat. By roasting fiber-rich chickpeas in heavenly spices you can create a snack that satisfies food cravings and provides the necessary crunch we all love.

1   Preheat the oven to 400°F. Line a baking sheet with parchment paper. Set aside.

2   Combine all of the ingredients and mix well.

3   Spread the chickpeas in a single layer on the prepared baking sheet. Roast for about 30–45 minutes until chickpeas are crispy.

EXCHANGES/ CHOICES		
1 Starch	Calories **80**	Sodium **185 mg**
	Calories from Fat **20**	Total Carbohydrate **11 g**
	Total Fat **2.5 g**	Dietary Fiber **3 g**
	Saturated Fat **0.3 g**	Sugars **2 g**
	Trans Fat **0.0 g**	Protein **3 g**
	Cholesterol **0 mg**	

Quickie Cream Cheese Dips

Start with 8 ounces low-fat cream cheese or Neufchatel cheese and make one of the following dips:

CLAM DIP

To the 8 ounces of cheese, add 1/2 cup minced onion; 1 garlic clove, minced; 1 teaspoon fresh lemon juice; 1 teaspoon grated horseradish; and 6 ounces minced canned clams. Blend well and serve.

CHUTNEY DIP

To the 8 ounces of cheese, add 1/2 bottle spicy chutney. Blend well, place in a bowl, sprinkle with chopped scallions, and serve.

TUNA DIP

To the 8 ounces of cheese, add 7 ounces water-packed, flaked, canned tuna; juice of half a lemon; 1/2 minced onion, and 2 tablespoons minced fresh basil. Blend well and serve.

Sausage Stuffed Mushrooms

18 large cremini mushrooms

3/4 cup plain dry bread crumbs, divided

2 tablespoons grated Parmesan cheese

2 ounces chicken sausage links, casings removed

1 large onion, finely chopped

1 small red bell pepper, finely chopped

2 tablespoons fresh minced parsley

1/4 teaspoon pepper

Stuffed mushrooms are always a hit at cocktail parties, but they can also be laden with grease and calorie dense. Not these! Go ahead and nibble away.

1   Preheat oven to 400°F. Remove stems from mushrooms and finely chop stems. Mix 2 tablespoons bread crumbs and Parmesan in small bowl.

2   Lightly coat large nonstick skillet with nonstick cooking spray and set over medium heat. Cook sausages until they begin to brown, about 5 minutes, breaking up with side of spoon. Stir in onion, red pepper, mushroom stems, and parsley and cook until vegetables are soft, about 5 minutes. Stir in remaining bread crumbs and black pepper. Remove from heat. Add 1 teaspoon of water at a time until you have a stuffing that is moist enough to mound.

3   Mound stuffing in mushrooms and arrange, stuffing-side up, in 13 × 9-inch baking dish. Sprinkle with Parmesan mixture. Bake until heated through, about 9 minutes.

EXCHANGES/ CHOICES		
1 Starch 1 Vegetable 1/2 Fat	Calories **115** Calories from Fat **25** Total Fat **3.0 g** Saturated Fat **1.0 g** Trans Fat **0.0 g** Cholesterol **10 mg**	Sodium **195 mg** Total Carbohydrate **17 g** Dietary Fiber **2 g** Sugars **4 g** Protein **6 g**

Spanish Style Dates With Bacon, p. 13

Spanish Style Dates with Bacon

20 pitted large dates

20 roasted, unsalted almonds

10 slices bacon, cut crosswise in half

This may be short on ingredients, but three powerfully flavorful ingredients are all you need for a spectacular appetizer. The sweetness of the dates, crunch of the almonds, and the smoky bacon all come together into one fantastic mouthful.

1 Preheat oven to 400°F. Cut a small slit in each date. Insert an almond into the date and press the date together to seal. Wrap each date with a bacon slice.

2 Line a baking sheet with foil or parchment paper. Place a roasting rack on top of the baking sheet. Add the dates and roast for 20 minutes until the dates are hot and the bacon is crisp. Serve immediately with toothpicks.

EXCHANGES/ CHOICES	Calories **45** Calories from Fat **20**	Sodium **70 mg**
1/2 Fruit 1/2 Fat	Total Fat **2.0 g** Saturated Fat **0.5 g** Trans Fat **0.0 g** Cholesterol **5 mg**	Total Carbohydrate **6 g** Dietary Fiber **1 g** Sugars **5 g** Protein **2 g**

Savory Ginger Beef BBQ Appetizer

1 pound boneless lean
   sirloin tip roast or sirloin
   steak

2 tablespoons oyster sauce

2 scallions, finely minced

4 garlic cloves, finely
   minced

1 tablespoon hoisin sauce

2 teaspoons toasted
   sesame oil

2 teaspoons fresh grated
   ginger

1 teaspoon liquid smoke

1/4 teaspoon sugar

freshly ground black
   pepper, to taste

Little nibbles like these will have your guests coming back for more. Combining so many elements of flavor—sweet, salty, and spicy—this appetizer will outshine the usual fare that is served. When this many flavors combine, you have the ultimate comfort food.

1 Cut the beef into 1-inch cubes and place in a medium-sized bowl.

2 Combine the remaining ingredients in a separate bowl and add to the beef. Marinate, covered, for at least 1 hour or overnight in the refrigerator.

3 When ready to cook, coat a grill pan with cooking spray. Add the beef and cook about 2 minutes per side or until desired doneness. Spear with a toothpick to serve. Discard marinade.

EXCHANGES/
CHOICES

2 Lean Meat

Calories **80**
   Calories from Fat **25**

Total Fat **3.0 g**
   Saturated Fat **0.9 g**
   Trans Fat **0.1 g**

Cholesterol **20 mg**

Sodium **110 mg**

Total Carbohydrate **1 g**
   Dietary Fiber **0 g**
   Sugars **1 g**

Protein **11 g**

Sweet Onion, White Bean, and Artichoke Dip

2 tablespoons olive oil

1 small Vidalia or other sweet onion, chopped

1 1/2 teaspoons sugar

4 garlic cloves, minced

1 15-ounce can cannellini beans, drained and rinsed

2 tablespoons fresh lemon juice

1 teaspoon dried oregano

1 teaspoon dried basil

pinch cayenne

sea salt, to taste

freshly ground black pepper, to taste

1 15-ounce can artichoke hearts in water, drained

1/4 cup rehydrated diced sun-dried tomatoes

Who knew that by combining beans and artichoke hearts you could easily simulate the taste of a full-fat party dip? By caramelizing the sweet onion, you add a bit of sweetness to the earthier flavors of the beans and artichokes. Adding sun-dried tomatoes gives attractive bits of color and taste.

1   Heat the oil in a skillet over medium-high heat. Add the onion, sugar, and garlic and sauté for 5 minutes.

2   Add the mixture to a blender or food processor. Add the remaining ingredients and purée until smooth, but thick.

EXCHANGES/ CHOICES	Calories **40**	Sodium **80 mg**
	Calories from Fat **15**	Total Carbohydrate **5 g**
1/2 Carbohydrate	Total Fat **1.5 g**	Dietary Fiber **1 g**
	Saturated Fat **0.2 g**	Sugars **1 g**
	Trans Fat **0.0 g**	Protein **2 g**
	Cholesterol **0 mg**	

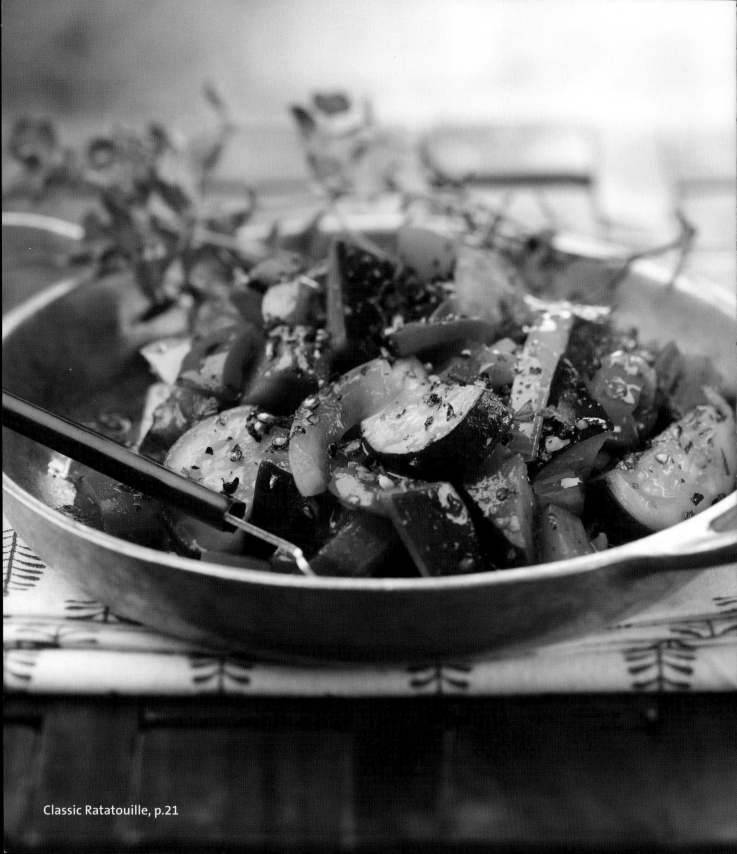

Classic Ratatouille, p.21

CHAPTER 2
Sides and Salads

Apple and Gorgonzola Cheese Salad | 18

Braised Cabbage and Apples | 19

Caesar Salad with Chicken | 20

Classic Ratatouille | 21

Chopped Salad with Cilantro Lime Dressing | 22

Creamy Polenta | 24

Creamy Succotash | 25

Crispy Roasted Cauliflower | 26

Ginger Carrots with Golden Raisins and Lemon | 27

Greek Country Salad | 28

Maple Apples | 29

Parmesan Popovers | 30

Roasted Potatoes, Carrots, and Parsnips | 31

Rustic Garlic and Olive Oil Mashed Potatoes | 32

Saffron Asparagus Risotto with Peas | 33

Spaghetti Squash with Pine Nuts and Sage | 35

Spiced Sweet Potato Wedges | 36

Spinach with Golden Raisins | 37

Steamed New Potatoes with Creamy Herb Dressing | 38

Sweet Potato and Squash Mash | 39

Tomato, Basil, and Mozzarella Salad | 40

Apple and Gorgonzola Cheese Salad

SALAD

2 large (8 ounces each) Braeburn apples, thinly sliced

2 tablespoons fresh lemon juice

1 large carrot, peeled and thinly sliced

8 cups mixed salad greens

1 small red onion, thinly sliced

VINAIGRETTE

2 tablespoons fresh orange juice

2 tablespoons fresh lemon juice

1 tablespoon honey

2 teaspoons Dijon mustard

1/4 cup walnut oil

sea salt, to taste

freshly ground black pepper, to taste

GARNISH

1/4 cup toasted walnut pieces

3 tablespoons crumbled Gorgonzola cheese

You wouldn't necessarily think of a salad as comfort food, but when it's got Gorgonzola, declare the salad soothing! Pairing tart fall Braeburn apples with fresh citrus flavors and earthy walnut oil, this salad may appear on your dinner table more often than you think.

1 Coat the apples with the lemon juice and set aside. Place the carrot slices and mixed greens on a platter. Top with the onion and set aside.

2 Whisk together the orange and lemon juices, honey, and mustard. Slowly add the oil in a thin stream, whisking constantly.

3 Add the apples to the salad. Top with walnuts and cheese. Drizzle on the vinaigrette.

EXCHANGES/ CHOICES		
	Calories **150**	Sodium **95 mg**
	Calories from Fat **90**	Total Carbohydrate **14 g**
1 Fruit	Total Fat **10.0 g**	Dietary Fiber **3 g**
2 Fat	Saturated Fat **1.5 g**	Sugars **10 g**
	Trans Fat **0.0 g**	Protein **2 g**
	Cholesterol **0 mg**	

Braised Cabbage and Apples

2 teaspoons vegetable oil

1 small onion, finely chopped

1 teaspoon caraway seeds

1 pound green cabbage, cored and thinly sliced (6 1/2 cups)

1 tablespoon cider vinegar

salt, to taste

2 small (3 ounces each) crisp red apples (such as Gala, Braeburn, or Empire), cored and cut into small cubes

1 teaspoon honey

2 tablespoons chopped walnuts, toasted (optional)

Cabbage is such a part of my Eastern European heritage; it always showed up on the dinner plate when we needed a little comfort food. What I love most about cabbage is how long it stores and still cooks up with great flavor.

1   Heat oil in large skillet over medium heat. Add onion and caraway seeds. Sauté until onion is softened, about 5 minutes.

2   Stir in cabbage, vinegar, and salt. Cover. Cook just until cabbage wilts, about 4 minutes. Uncover. Increase heat to high. Add apples and honey. Cook, stirring frequently, until apples are crisp-tender and most of liquid cooks off, about 4 to 6 minutes. Transfer to a serving plate. Top with walnuts, if desired, and serve.

EXCHANGES/ CHOICES		
1/2 Carbohydrate	Calories **25**	Sodium **5 mg**
	Calories from Fat **10**	Total Carbohydrate **5 g**
	Total Fat **1.0 g**	Dietary Fiber **1 g**
	Saturated Fat **0.1 g**	Sugars **3 g**
	Trans Fat **0.0 g**	Protein **1 g**
	Cholesterol **0 mg**	

Choosing the Right Cooking Oil

When making salads and preparing vegetables, it is often confusing to know which cooking oil is appropriate for each dish. Here is a quick cheat sheet for choosing the correct oil for various cooking methods and situations.

EXTRA VIRGIN OLIVE OIL

Use for virtually all cold salad dressings and light sautéing.

CANOLA OIL

Use when you want the oil flavor to be less dominant than olive oil. It is also good for sautéing and stir-frying.

PEANUT OIL

Use for all stir-frying. High heat, high smoke point, and excellent flavor make this an excellent choice for Asian cooking.

AROMATIC NUT OILS (LIKE WALNUT OR HAZELNUT)

Use nut oils to lightly drizzle over cooked vegetables or salads.

SESAME OIL

Drizzle on Asian flavored foods and use in some Asian style sauces and dips.

Caesar Salad with Chicken*

1–1 1/2 pounds boneless, skinless chicken breasts or meatless chicken strips or patties

4–5 tablespoons olive oil, divided

1/4 teaspoon salt

1/8 teaspoon garlic powder

2 large (about 1 1/4 ounces each) slices sourdough bread, cut into 1/2-inch cubes (or buy packaged croutons)

1/4 teaspoon kosher salt

2 tablespoons reduced-fat mayonnaise

1/2 teaspoon minced garlic

2 tablespoons fresh lemon juice

1 teaspoon Worcestershire sauce

1/2 teaspoon anchovy paste, or use mashed capers

1 head romaine lettuce, washed, dried, and cut or ripped into bite-sized pieces (8–10 cups)

1/4 cup shredded Parmesan cheese

* Recipe courtesy of Aviva Goldfarb and her daughter Celia

I had to include a classic Caesar Salad recipe in this book and you can adapt the recipe to suit your family's palate. Vegetarians can use meatless chicken strips or patties instead of the chicken breasts, you can also use shrimp, or you can even leave the protein out completely and serve it as a side dish. Serve with fresh warmed whole-grain bread.

1 Preheat the oven or toaster oven to 400°F if you are making your own croutons.

2 Cut each chicken breast crosswise into thin strips. Place the chicken in a flat dish, drizzle with 1 tablespoon oil, salt, and the garlic powder, and flip the chicken several times to coat it. Heat a large nonstick skillet over medium heat. Sauté the chicken, turning occasionally, until it is cooked through, 5–7 minutes.

3 To make the croutons, in a medium bowl, toss the bread cubes with 1–2 tablespoons oil and the kosher salt. Place them on a baking sheet in a single layer and bake them in the preheated oven for 3–5 minutes, until they are slightly crisp and browned. Watch them carefully so they don't burn. Set them aside.

4 To make the dressing, thoroughly whisk together the mayonnaise, 2 tablespoons olive oil, minced garlic, lemon juice, Worcestershire sauce, and anchovy paste.

5 Just before serving, vigorously toss the lettuce, cheese, chicken, croutons, and dressing in a large salad bowl.

EXCHANGES/ CHOICES
1/2 Carbohydrate
2 Lean Meat
1/2 Fat

Calories 145
Calories from Fat 65
Total Fat 7.0 g
Saturated Fat 1.5 g
Trans Fat 0.0 g
Cholesterol 35 mg

Sodium 210 mg
Total Carbohydrate 5 g
Dietary Fiber 1 g
Sugars 1 g
Protein 14 g

Classic Ratatouille

1 small eggplant, unpeeled, top removed

1/4 teaspoon salt

3 tablespoons olive oil, divided

1 onion, thickly sliced

1 small green pepper, seeded and chopped

1 small red pepper, seeded and chopped

2 garlic cloves, minced

4 medium tomatoes, seeded and coarsely chopped

2 small zucchini, halved lengthwise and cut crosswise into 1/2-inch strips

1/4 teaspoon dried thyme

1/4 teaspoon dried oregano

1/4–1/2 teaspoon freshly ground black pepper

1/8 teaspoon cayenne

Ratatouille is the ultimate comfort food in France. Although perhaps not thought of as a comfort food here in the U.S., it should be! A rich stewed mixture of fresh garden vegetables is so satisfying any time of year. I make mine with a lot less fat than the traditional recipe, keeping it light and fresh. But it still packs a flavorful punch!

1   Cut the eggplant into 3/4-inch cubes. Place the eggplant in a colander and sprinkle it with salt. Place a heavy bowl over the eggplant and let stand for 1/2 hour.

2   In a large skillet or Dutch oven, heat 1 tablespoon of the oil on medium-high heat. Add the onion and red and green peppers and sauté for 5 minutes. Add the garlic and tomatoes and sauté for 3 minutes. Remove the mixture from the pan and set aside.

3   Heat 1 tablespoon of oil and add the zucchini to the skillet. Sauté on medium-high heat for about 10 minutes. Remove the zucchini and place with the other vegetables.

4   Rinse the salt from the eggplant and dry it with a paper towel. Add 1 tablespoon of oil to the skillet. Sauté the eggplant on medium heat for 6–7 minutes. Add the reserved vegetables to the eggplant. Stir in the thyme, oregano, pepper, and cayenne and cook for 5 minutes.

EXCHANGES/ CHOICES		
3 Vegetable 2 Fat	Calories **185** Calories from Fat **100** Total Fat **11.0 g** Saturated Fat **1.5 g** Trans Fat **0.0 g** Cholesterol **0 mg**	Sodium **15 mg** Total Carbohydrate **22 g** Dietary Fiber **6 g** Sugars **10 g** Protein **4 g**

Chopped Salad with Cilantro Lime Dressing

SALAD

4 cups thinly sliced romaine lettuce

2 carrots, peeled and diced

2 celery stalks, diced

2 plum tomatoes, seeded and diced

1/2 cup peeled and diced cucumber

1 cup canned black beans, drained

DRESSING

2 tablespoons cider vinegar

2 tablespoons fresh lime juice

2 tablespoons chopped cilantro

2 teaspoons honey

1/2 teaspoon sea salt

1/4 teaspoon black pepper

1/4 cup olive oil

3 tablespoons toasted pumpkin or sunflower seeds

Instead of a tossed salad, try something new and different. Rows of salad ingredients make for a pretty presentation and it's easy to identify exactly what you're eating. The cilantro dressing is so sublime; pour it over any other green salad to make that salad shine.

1 Place the lettuce on a shallow platter. In rows, arrange the carrots, celery, plum tomatoes, cucumber, and black beans.

2 Prepare the salad dressing. Whisk together the cider vinegar, lime juice, cilantro, honey, salt, and pepper. Slowly drizzle in the oil, whisking to incorporate.

3 Drizzle on the dressing. Top with toasted pumpkin or sunflower seeds.

EXCHANGES/ CHOICES		
1/2 Starch	Calories **140**	Sodium **210 mg**
1 Vegetable	Calories from Fat **80**	Total Carbohydrate **11 g**
1 1/2 Fat	Total Fat **9.0 g**	Dietary Fiber **4 g**
	Saturated Fat **1.4 g**	Sugars **4 g**
	Trans Fat **0.0 g**	Protein **4 g**
	Cholesterol **0 mg**	

Chopped Salad with Cilantro Lime Dressing, p. 22

Creamy Polenta

4 cups water

1 cup coarse ground yellow polenta

1 tablespoon mascarpone cheese

2 tablespoons freshly grated Parmesan cheese

sea salt, to taste

freshly ground black pepper, to taste

I served this polenta to my Italian friends who thought I got this recipe from one of their relatives! When I told them there is not one scrap of butter in it, they refused to believe me. This creamy side dish has a double life when transformed into crispy croutons. The versatility of polenta never ceases to amaze me.

1 In a 2-quart saucepan bring the water to a boil. Slowly add the polenta, whisking constantly. (Do not add the polenta all at once as it will sit in one large mass and will be difficult to stir.) Continue to whisk over medium heat until the mixture looks thick, but is still creamy and starts to pull away from the sides of the pan, about 10–15 minutes. You may need to switch to a wooden spoon to stir.

2 Remove the pot from heat. Whisk in the cheeses. Season with salt and pepper and serve immediately.

EXCHANGES/ CHOICES		
1 Starch	Calories **80** Calories from Fat **15** Total Fat **1.5 g** Saturated Fat **0.8 g** Trans Fat **0.0 g** Cholesterol **5 mg**	Sodium **20 mg** Total Carbohydrate **14 g** Dietary Fiber **1 g** Sugars **0 g** Protein **2 g**

Variation: Polenta Croutons

SERVES 14
SERVING SIZE 6–7 croutons

1 Preheat the oven to 350°F. Prepare Creamy Polenta and pour it into an 8 × 8-inch glass pan, cover, and refrigerate overnight. Turn the polenta onto a cutting board and cut into 1/2 × 1/2-inch cubes. Toss the croutons in a bowl with olive oil cooking spray and 1 teaspoon Italian dry seasoning to coat.

2 Spread the croutons in a single layer on a baking sheet. Bake them for 1 hour until dry and toasted.

EXCHANGES/ CHOICES				
1/2 Starch	Calories **45** Calories from Fat **10**	Total Fat **1.0 g** Saturated Fat **0.5 g** Trans Fat **0.0 g**	Cholesterol **0 mg** Sodium **8 mg**	Total Carbohydrate **0 g** Dietary Fiber **0 g** Sugars **0 g** Protein **1 g**

Creamy Succotash*

2 cups fresh or frozen baby lima beans

2 cups fresh corn kernels

1 cup fat-free half-and-half

1 tablespoon light olive oil

kosher salt, to taste

3 tablespoons chopped fresh chives

1/4 teaspoon freshly ground black pepper

Steamed vegetables are nice, but for true classic comfort, there is nothing like a creamy succotash. The chives at the end lift the entire dish with almost a spring-like finish.

1 Bring lima beans, corn, half-and-half, olive oil, and salt to boil in large saucepan over high heat.

2 Reduce heat to medium, cover, and cook until tender, 10–12 minutes. Remove from heat and stir in chives and pepper.

*Adapted from *Eat To Beat Diabetes* (Readers Digest, 2007)

EXCHANGES/ CHOICES		
1/2 Starch 1/2 Fat	Calories **105** Calories from Fat **20** Total Fat **2.5 g** Saturated Fat **0.6 g** Trans Fat **0.0 g** Cholesterol **0 mg**	Sodium **60 mg** Total Carbohydrate **18 g** Dietary Fiber **3 g** Sugars **3 g** Protein **4 g**

5 Great Salad Add-Ins

1. FRESH HERBS AS GREENS.

Fresh basil, sorrel, dill, thyme, and oregano are delicious when added to any salad.

2. REHYDRATED SLICED SUN-DRIED TOMATOES.

Toss in a few for a highlight in every bite.

3. DICED ROASTED RED OR YELLOW PEPPERS.

Excellent all by themselves, drizzled with a little olive oil, salt, and pepper.

4. PARMESAN CHEESE (SHREDDED OR IN SHARDS).

Spike any salad with just a little bit of this prized cheese.

5. SLICED JICAMA, JERUSALEM ARTICHOKES, AND FENNEL SLICES.

All add exotic accents to any salad.

Crispy Roasted Cauliflower

1 medium head
cauliflower, cut into
small florets

2 teaspoons olive oil

kosher salt, to taste

freshly ground black
pepper, to taste

TOPPING

1/2 cup fresh breadcrumbs
(preferably made from
Italian bread)

1 tablespoon freshly
grated Parmesan cheese

2 teaspoons olive oil

1/2 teaspoon dried
oregano

Simply prepared vegetables are often the tastiest and most satisfying part of a meal. In this case, less is really more. My guests couldn't believe that I made this dish with so few ingredients.

1 Preheat the oven to 425°F. Line a 10 × 15-inch baking sheet with parchment paper.

2 Bring a 2-quart pot of water to a boil. Add the cauliflower, turn off the heat and let the cauliflower stand in the water for 2 minutes. Drain the cauliflower into a colander and place it in a single layer on a kitchen towel. Pat the cauliflower dry with another kitchen towel and allow it to sit for 5 minutes to dry thoroughly. This helps ensure the crispness as they roast in the oven.

3 Add the cauliflower to a bowl. Toss the cauliflower with 2 teaspoons olive oil, salt, and pepper.

4 Mix the breadcrumbs, Parmesan cheese, 2 teaspoons of olive oil, and dried oregano in a small bowl. Add mixture to the cauliflower and toss well with tongs.

5 Spread the cauliflower onto the prepared pan in a single layer. Roast for about 20–25 minutes until the cauliflower is crispy but not overcooked, and the breadcrumbs are browned. To ensure crispness, allow the cauliflower to rest for 5 minutes on the baking sheet before serving.

EXCHANGES/ CHOICES		
1 Vegetable 1/2 Fat	Calories **50** Calories from Fat **25** Total Fat **3.0 g** Saturated Fat **0.5 g** Trans Fat **0.0 g** Cholesterol **0 mg**	Sodium **50 mg** Total Carbohydrate **5 g** Dietary Fiber **2 g** Sugars **1 g** Protein **2 g**

Ginger Carrots with Golden Raisins and Lemon

1/2 cup golden or black raisins

5 medium carrots

2 teaspoons finely minced fresh ginger

juice of 1/2 lemon

2 teaspoons butter

2 teaspoons brown sugar

2 teaspoons cornstarch

1 teaspoon grated lemon zest

Remember very sweet glazed carrots? Here they are delightfully sweet but without that thick, heavy sauce. The lemon really makes this dish shine with a lovely vibrancy.

1 Bring 3 cups water to a boil in a medium saucepan.

2 Meanwhile, in a medium bowl, combine the raisins and hot water. Cover. Let stand for about 15 minutes.

3 Meanwhile, peel and slice the carrots diagonally into 1/2-inch pieces. In a large pot of boiling water, add the carrots, ginger, and lemon juice. Cook the carrots for about 6 to 7 minutes. Drain.

4 Drain the raisins, reserving 3/4–cup liquid and set aside. In a skillet, melt the butter over medium heat. Add the brown sugar and cook 30 seconds. Mix together the reserved raisin water and cornstarch. Add to the butter brown sugar mixture. Cook for about 1 minute, until thickened. Add the raisins and carrots and cook for 1 minute. Add the lemon zest and serve.

EXCHANGES/ CHOICES		
1 Fruit	Calories **115**	Sodium **70 mg**
2 Vegetable	Calories from Fat **20**	Total Carbohydrate **25 g**
1/2 Fat	Total Fat **2.0 g**	Dietary Fiber **3 g**
	Saturated Fat **1.3 g**	Sugars **17 g**
	Trans Fat **0.0 g**	Protein **1 g**
	Cholesterol **5 mg**	

Greek Country Salad

1/2 medium red onion, thinly sliced

2 tomatoes, cut into wedges

1 yellow bell pepper, cut into thin strips

1/2 English cucumber, cut into thin slices

DRESSING

1 1/2 tablespoons olive oil

2 teaspoons fresh lemon juice

2 teaspoons dried oregano

sea salt, to taste

freshly ground black pepper, to taste

GARNISH

1/4 cup pitted Kalamata olives

3 tablespoons reduced-fat feta cheese

To me, one of the most comforting cuisines in the world is Greek. One of my very favorite salads is a Greek salad. This version, direct from my travels through Greece, is more streamlined than the ones served in the U.S. I think you will love its straightforwardness; just fresh veggies enhanced with a little olive oil and a sprinkling of creamy feta.

1 Toss the red onion, tomatoes, pepper, and cucumber together.

2 Whisk the olive oil, lemon juice, oregano, salt, and pepper.

3 Drizzle the dressing over vegetables and top with olives and feta cheese.

EXCHANGES/ CHOICES		
2 Vegetable 1 1/2 Fat	Calories **105** Calories from Fat **65** Total Fat **7.0 g** Saturated Fat **1.4 g** Trans Fat **0.0 g** Cholesterol **0 mg**	Sodium **160 mg** Total Carbohydrate **10 g** Dietary Fiber **2 g** Sugars **4 g** Protein **3 g**

5 Steps to Making a Perfect Salad

1. Select a mixture of different greens for better nutrition and contrasting textures and flavors.

2. Tear the leaves with your hands rather than cutting the leaves, to avoid bruising the delicate leaves.

3. Prepare your dressing at least 1/2 hour prior to serving so the flavors can meld.

4. Add the salad dressing to the bowl. Add the greens and toss gently to coat the leaves. Use less dressing than you think; dressing should just lightly coat the greens.

5. Add salt and pepper to the salad at the last moment. Adding salt and pepper earlier causes the greens to wilt.

Maple Apples

2 Granny Smith or Braeburn apples, unpeeled and sliced into 1/2-inch wedges

1 tablespoon fresh lemon juice

1 teaspoon canola oil

1/4 cup apple cider

1 tablespoon pure maple syrup

1/4 teaspoon cinnamon

1/4 teaspoon ground cloves

1 tablespoon toasted slivered almonds

Do you love apple pie, but don't have time to make a crust? Why not use the same flavors commonly found in an apple pie, without the crust? You can serve this alongside a grilled pork entrée, or top it with a scoop of reduced-fat ice cream or frozen yogurt for a delicious dessert. The best part: it takes less than 30 minutes to make.

1 In a small bowl, toss the apples with the lemon juice.

2 Heat the oil in a large skillet over medium heat. Add the apples and sauté for 6 minutes, or until the apples develop a rich brown color. Reduce the heat to low, cover, and cool for 3 minutes until apples are soft. Remove the apples with a slotted spoon and set aside.

3 In the same skillet, add the remaining ingredients except the almonds. Bring to a boil and cook over medium heat until syrupy. Add the apples and sprinkle with the almonds.

EXCHANGES/ CHOICES		
1 Fruit	Calories **80**	Sodium **0 mg**
1/2 Fat	Calories from Fat **20**	Total Carbohydrate **16 g**
	Total Fat **2.5 g**	Dietary Fiber **2 g**
	Saturated Fat **0.2 g**	Sugars **12 g**
	Trans Fat **0.0 g**	Protein **1 g**
	Cholesterol **0 mg**	

Parmesan Popovers

1 cup all-purpose flour, sifted

1/4 cup plus 1 tablespoon freshly grated Parmesan cheese

pinch salt

1/4 teaspoon freshly ground black pepper

2 large eggs

1 egg white

1 cup 1% milk

1 tablespoon butter, melted

2 scallions, minced (white and green part)

As much as I know about food science, it never ceases to amaze me the rising power of a popover. I'm like an excited little kid when I see the popovers grow tall. It's refreshing to get so excited about food, isn't it?

1 Preheat oven to 425°F. Lightly coat 12-cup popover pan or muffin tin with nonstick cooking spray and put in oven to preheat. Whisk flour, Parmesan, salt, and pepper in medium bowl. Make a well in center of flour mixture.

2 Whisk eggs, egg white, milk, and butter until frothy. Pour into well of flour mixture and whisk just until smooth. Stir in scallions.

3 When a drop of water dances and sizzles in the pan, it's hot enough. Spoon in batter, dividing it evenly among the 12 cups. Bake 15 minutes. Reduce oven temperature to 350°F and bake until golden and puffed, about 10 minutes longer. Immediately remove popovers from pan and quickly make a small slit in the side of each to release steam.

EXCHANGES/ CHOICES	Calories **80**	Sodium **50 mg**
	Calories from Fat **25**	Total Carbohydrate **9 g**
1/2 Starch	Total Fat **3.0 g**	Dietary Fiber **0 g**
1/2 Fat	Saturated Fat **1.4 g**	Sugars **1 g**
	Trans Fat **0.0 g**	Protein **4 g**
	Cholesterol **40 mg**	

Roasted Potatoes, Carrots, and Parsnips

5 large (2 3/4 ounces each) carrots, peeled, ends trimmed, sliced on diagonal

4 large (5 ounces each) parsnips, peeled, ends trimmed, sliced on diagonal

2 (5 ounces each) sweet potatoes, peeled, cut into medium cubes

2 tablespoons olive oil

1 teaspoon kosher salt

2 tablespoons fresh herbs (thyme, oregano, sage, or rosemary)

freshly ground black pepper, to taste

When everyone else was bringing sweet potatoes capped with marshmallows to holiday dinners, our family would bring this lovely roasted mixture of potatoes, carrots, and parsnips. The technique of roasting is actually the comforting part; the high temperature puts a crispy crust on root vegetables that beats sweet potatoes and marshmallows every time.

1 Heat the oven to 450°F. In a large bowl, combine the vegetables with the oil, salt, and herbs. Toss to coat.

2 Arrange vegetables on two parchment paper–lined baking sheets. Roast until soft on the inside and browned on the outside, about 20–30 minutes. Flip the vegetables halfway through the cooking.

3 Serve warm or at room temperature.

EXCHANGES/ CHOICES		
1 Starch 1/2 Fat	Calories **90**	Sodium **230 mg**
	Calories from Fat **25**	Total Carbohydrate **16 g**
	Total Fat **3.0 g**	Dietary Fiber **3 g**
	Saturated Fat **0.4 g**	Sugars **5 g**
	Trans Fat **0.0 g**	Protein **1 g**
	Cholesterol **0 mg**	

Rustic Garlic and Olive Oil Mashed Potatoes

2 pounds peeled and halved russet potatoes

14 peeled, whole garlic cloves

3 1/2 tablespoons olive oil

1/3 cup grated fresh Parmesan cheese

kosher salt, to taste

freshly ground black pepper, to taste

Mashed potatoes go Italian! Italians eat mashed potatoes, perhaps not in the profuse amounts that we do in America, but their mashed potatoes are heavy on flavor. Mashing them with 14, yes that's right, 14 garlic cloves, makes for unbelievable flavor. By using olive oil instead of butter, the nutritional value is increased. Although a lot of low-fat mashed potato recipes call for using chicken stock in place of cream or milk, I find that the broth actually dilutes the flavor of the potatoes. All you need is some of the cooking liquid and the olive oil to give the potatoes body and creaminess.

1   Bring a large pot of salted water to a boil. Add the potatoes and garlic and bring to boil. Lower the heat, cover, and simmer on low heat for about 25–35 minutes or until very tender.

2   Drain the potatoes, saving 1/2 cup of the cooking liquid. Add the potatoes back to the pot. Place a dishtowel over the pan and cover. Let the potatoes dry steam for 5 minutes.

3   Slowly add the cooking liquid to the potatoes, mashing well. Add the olive oil and continue to mash the potatoes to desired consistency. Add in the Parmesan cheese, salt, and pepper.

EXCHANGES/ CHOICES		
1 Starch 1 1/2 Fat	Calories **150** Calories from Fat **65**	Sodium **35 mg** Total Carbohydrate **19 g** Dietary Fiber **2 g** Sugars **1 g** Protein **3 g**
	Total Fat **7.0 g** Saturated Fat **1.5 g** Trans Fat **0.0 g** Cholesterol **5 mg**	

Saffron Asparagus Risotto with Peas

9 cups low-fat, reduced-sodium chicken broth

large pinch saffron threads

2 small sprigs rosemary

2 sprigs thyme

1 tablespoon garlic oil (or olive oil)

1 large onion, diced

1 large leek, washed and bottom thinly sliced (about 2 cups)

3 cloves garlic, minced

2 1/2 cups Arborio rice

sea salt, to taste

freshly ground pepper, to taste

1 cup dry white wine (Pinot Grigio is best)

1 cup asparagus, thinly sliced on the diagonal

1 cup frozen peas

1/2 cup dry-packed sun-dried tomatoes, rehydrated and sliced

1/4 cup fresh chopped basil

1/4 cup fresh Parmesan or Pecorino Romano cheese (optional)

2 teaspoons fresh lemon zest

Saffron's rich golden color enhances this creamy dish. With so many versions of this classic Italian comfort food, this one is beautiful, lower in fat and calories, and simple to make.

1 Heat the broth in a medium pot over medium heat. Crumble in the saffron threads and stir to dissolve. Tie the rosemary and thyme in cheesecloth to make an herb sachet that will flavor the broth. Or, if you don't have cheesecloth, add the rosemary and thyme sprigs directly to the broth; just make sure you do not add them into the rice mixture.

2 Heat the oil in a large skillet or a wide, shallow stockpot, over medium heat. Add the onion, leek, and garlic, cover, and cook for 3 minutes. Add the rice and sauté uncovered for 5 minutes. Season with salt and pepper. Add the wine to the rice and cook until the rice absorbs the liquid, constantly stirring in a circular motion.

3 Add two ladlefuls of broth to the rice and stir until the liquid is absorbed. Keep adding a ladleful at a time to the rice until the last ladleful is added and the rice is creamy. This entire process takes about 20 minutes. The risotto should be creamy.

4 Meanwhile, add the asparagus and peas to a microwave-safe container. Pour the remaining cup of chicken broth on top. Cover and microwave for about 6 minutes, just until vegetables are tender, but retain color. Drain the vegetables and set aside.

5 During the last 5 minutes of stirring, add in the asparagus, peas, sun-dried tomatoes, and the basil. Stir for 1 minute. Add the freshly grated cheese and lemon zest.

EXCHANGES/ CHOICES		
1 Starch	Calories **95**	Sodium **205 mg**
	Calories from Fat **5**	Total Carbohydrate **18 g**
	Total Fat **0.5 g**	Dietary Fiber **1 g**
	Saturated Fat **0.1 g**	Sugars **2 g**
	Trans Fat **0.0 g**	Protein **3 g**
	Cholesterol **0 mg**	

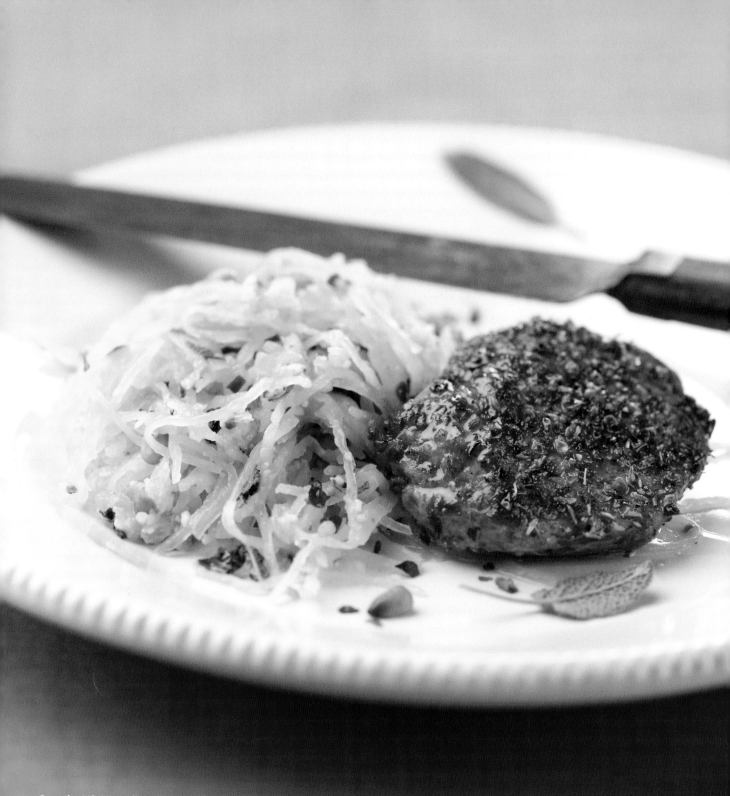

Spaghetti Squash with Pine Nuts and Sage, p. 35; Greek Lamb Chops, p. 99

Spaghetti Squash with Pine Nuts and Sage

1 medium (2 pounds) spaghetti squash, halved and seeded

2 teaspoons olive oil

1 onion, minced

1 large shallot, minced

2 garlic cloves, minced

1/4 cup pine nuts

2 tablespoons freshly grated Romano cheese

1 tablespoon minced fresh sage

1/4 teaspoon crushed red pepper flakes

sea salt, to taste

freshly ground pepper, to taste

I remember making my first spaghetti squash when I was a teenager. My sister and I had so much fun combing out strands of the squash as you would spaghetti. We always called spaghetti squash "our" spaghetti. This version is much more grown up with the flavors of sage and cheese, but to be honest, I could still top spaghetti squash with a little marinara sauce and call it a meal.

1   Preheat the oven to 400°F. Place the squash halves cut-side down on a parchment paper–lined baking sheet and roast for about 50 minutes, or until tender.

2   Meanwhile, heat the olive oil in a skillet over medium heat. Add the onion, shallot, and garlic and sauté for 4 minutes. Add in the pine nuts and cook for 2 minutes until the pine nuts are lightly browned. Set aside.

3   When the squash is cooked, turn over squash to cut side up. With a pasta rake or large spoon, scoop the flesh from the squash shell. The flesh will come out like strands of spaghetti. Add the squash to a large serving bowl and rake through the strands to keep them separated. Add in the pine nut mixture, cheese, sage, crushed red pepper flakes, salt, and pepper. Toss well and serve.

EXCHANGES/ CHOICES		
1/2 Starch	Calories **95**	Sodium **35 mg**
1 Fat	Calories from Fat **55**	Total Carbohydrate **9 g**
	Total Fat **6.0 g**	Dietary Fiber **2 g**
	Saturated Fat **0.8 g**	Sugars **3 g**
	Trans Fat **0.0 g**	Protein **2 g**
	Cholesterol **0 mg**	

Spiced Sweet Potato Wedges

6 medium (5 ounces each) sweet potatoes

1 1/2 tablespoons olive oil

2 teaspoons sugar

1/2 teaspoon ground cinnamon

1/2 teaspoon kosher salt

1/4 teaspoon freshly ground black pepper

1/4 teaspoon cayenne pepper

Sweet potato wedges have more vitamin A, less fat, and fewer calories than any regular fries could hope to have. The beautiful burnt orange color and deep-spiced aromas make these really addictive, so keep your portions under control, but do enjoy!

1 Preheat the oven to 500°F.

2 Peel the potatoes and cut lengthwise into sixths. Combine the potatoes and the oil in a large bowl and toss well. Combine the sugar, cinnamon, salt, pepper, and cayenne pepper in a small bowl. Add the spice mixture to the potatoes and toss again.

3 Arrange the potatoes cut side down in a single layer on a baking sheet. Bake for 10 minutes. Turn the wedges over and bake 20 more minutes, until tender.

EXCHANGES/ CHOICES		
1/2 Starch 1/2 Fat	Calories **60** Calories from Fat **20** Total Fat **2.0 g** Saturated Fat **0.3 g** Trans Fat **0.0 g** Cholesterol **0 mg**	Sodium **95 mg** Total Carbohydrate **10 g** Dietary Fiber **2 g** Sugars **4 g** Protein **1 g**

Spinach with Golden Raisins

1/2 cup golden raisins

boiling water (to cover the raisins)

3 quarts water

2 pounds fresh spinach, washed, stemmed, and coarsely chopped

2 tablespoons olive oil

4 tablespoons pine nuts

4 garlic cloves, thickly sliced

kosher salt, to taste

freshly ground black pepper, to taste

This is a Sicilian recipe I learned in Italy many years ago. It's typically served at informal dinners. The added sweetness of the raisins tempers the peppery taste of spinach, so much that even finicky eaters will love this dish.

1 Place the raisins in a bowl with boiling water. Set aside for 10 minutes.

2 Meanwhile, bring the 3 quarts of water to a boil. Add the spinach a little at a time, pushing it down to the bottom of the pot with a spoon. Once all the spinach has been added, give it a good stir, and reduce the heat to medium-high and cook for 3 minutes. Drain and set aside.

3 Heat the olive oil, pine nuts, and garlic in a large skillet over medium heat and sauté for 2 minutes. Drain the raisins and discard the soaking water. Add the raisins and spinach to the pan and cook for 2 minutes. Season with salt and pepper.

EXCHANGES/ CHOICES		
1/2 Fruit	Calories **95**	Sodium **60 mg**
1 Vegetable	Calories from Fat **55**	Total Carbohydrate **10 g**
1 Fat	Total Fat **6.0 g**	Dietary Fiber **2 g**
	Saturated Fat **0.7 g**	Sugars **5 g**
	Trans Fat **0.0 g**	Protein **3 g**
	Cholesterol **0 mg**	

Choosing and Storing Fresh Greens

1. Select greens that are fresh, crisp, and vividly colored. Reject greens when you see insect damage or browning leaves.

2. Once home, discard wilted outer leaves and carefully wash the rest.

3. Dry the greens well by either method: dry on kitchen towels or in a salad spinner. Any wetness dilutes the dressing and reduces crispness.

4. Store the cleaned leaves in the refrigerator wrapped in a clean damp towel.

Steamed New Potatoes with Creamy Herb Dressing

1 pound new potatoes, scrubbed, halved

1/4 cup loosely packed fresh dill, stems removed

3/4 cup loosely packed parsley leaves, stems removed

2 tablespoons minced thyme

1/3 cup coarsely chopped chives

3/4 cup fat-free mayonnaise

1/2 cup low-fat buttermilk

2 tablespoons cider or champagne vinegar

3/4 teaspoon hot sauce

sea salt, to taste

freshly ground black pepper, to taste

My recipe testers unanimously agreed that they would prefer this creamy dressing to butter any day. Use the dressing separate from the potatoes to dress up steamed broccoli, asparagus, or a tossed salad. If you prefer a more robust dressing, add some rosemary or basil to the dressing as well. Do not substitute dried herbs for this dish; it simply won't work!

1   Fill the bottom of a large saucepan with 1 inch of water. Place a steamer rack inside the pot. Add the potatoes to the rack and cover. Steam the potatoes for about 15–17 minutes, until tender. Check on the water level and add more water if necessary. Test the tenderness of the potatoes by inserting a wooden or metal skewer into the potato. There should be no resistance.

2   While the potatoes steam, combine the dill, parsley, thyme, and chives with the mayonnaise in a food processor. Process until the herbs are chopped and are incorporated into the mayonnaise.

3   With the motor running, slowly pour the buttermilk through the feed tube and add in the vinegar, hot sauce, salt, and pepper. Process until combined. Adjust seasonings.

4   Serve the potatoes with the creamy herb dressing.

EXCHANGES/ CHOICES		
1 1/2 Starch	Calories **110**	Sodium **245 mg**
	Calories from Fat **10**	Total Carbohydrate **23 g**
	Total Fat **1.0 g**	Dietary Fiber **3 g**
	Saturated Fat **0.3 g**	Sugars **4 g**
	Trans Fat **0.0 g**	Protein **3 g**
	Cholesterol **5 mg**	

Sweet Potato and Squash Mash*

2 large (7 ounces each)
sweet potatoes

1/2 medium (1–2 pound)
butternut squash

1 ripe large banana

2 tablespoons brown sugar

1/2 tablespoon ground
cinnamon

A perfect fall side dish incorporating the best of the autumn harvest. The banana gives it a slight dessert-like panache.

1 Peel the sweet potatoes and cut into medium chunks. Discard any seeds from the butternut squash. Peel the squash and cut into medium chunks. Add the sweet potatoes and butternut squash to a large pot. Add water to cover and bring to a boil. Gently boil the potatoes and squash for about 30 minutes until fork tender.

2 Drain the squash and potatoes and add to a large bowl. Add the banana and mash with a potato masher until a creamy yet lumpy texture has developed.

3 Add the brown sugar and cinnamon and mix well.

*Recipe courtesy of
Corinne Dobbas, MS, RD

EXCHANGES/ CHOICES		
1 Starch 1/2 Fruit	Calories **100** Calories from Fat **0** Total Fat **0.0 g** Saturated Fat **0.1 g** Trans Fat **0.0 g** Cholesterol **0 mg**	Sodium **20 mg** Total Carbohydrate **25 g** Dietary Fiber **3 g** Sugars **11 g** Protein **1 g**

Tomato, Basil, and Mozzarella Salad

2 medium (5 ounces each) vine-ripened tomatoes

3 1/2 ounces part-skim mozzarella cheese

6 leaves fresh basil

2 teaspoons olive oil

sea salt, to taste

freshly ground black pepper, to taste

* Recipe courtesy of Alexandra Oppenheimer, RD

While we typically associate comfort foods with winter, this dish is a perfect complement to any summer meal.

1   Slice tomatoes into rounds and lay on a plate.

2   Slice the mozzarella into thin slices and place over each tomato.

3   Chop the basil and sprinkle evenly over the mozzarella.

4   Drizzle olive oil over all the slices and season with salt and pepper.

EXCHANGES/CHOICES

1 Fat

Calories **45**
Calories from Fat **25**
Total Fat **3.0 g**
Saturated Fat **1.4 g**
Trans Fat **0.0 g**
Cholesterol **10 mg**

Sodium **80 mg**
Total Carbohydrate **2 g**
Dietary Fiber **0 g**
Sugars **1 g**
Protein **3 g**

Make Your Own Flavored Vinegar

Make your salad dressing more appealing with homemade flavored vinegars! It's so easy. Just add a quart of cider or white wine vinegar to a 1-quart bottle. Add in one of the following variations, cap the bottle, and let the contents sit for a week before using. Drizzle on salads and vegetables with or without the addition of oil.

BASIL VINEGAR

Add 2 tablespoons dried basil, pinch sugar, 1/2 teaspoon minced garlic, 1 bay leaf, and 2 sprigs fresh oregano; add a few leaves fresh basil.

GARLIC VINEGAR

Add 3 cloves minced garlic; 2 garlic cloves, thinly sliced; and 5 whole peeled garlic cloves.

RASPBERRY VINEGAR

Add 1/2 cup mashed, frozen, unsweetened raspberries; pinch celery seeds; and 10 whole raspberries.

TARRAGON VINEGAR

Add 2 tablespoons dried tarragon, 1 peeled garlic clove, pinch sugar, and 1 large sprig fresh tarragon.

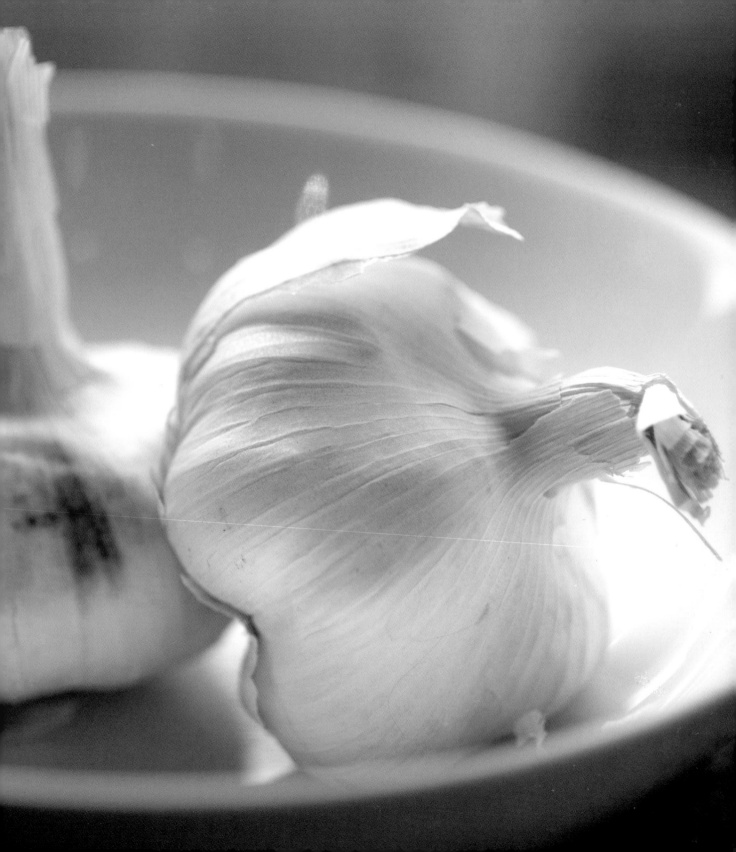

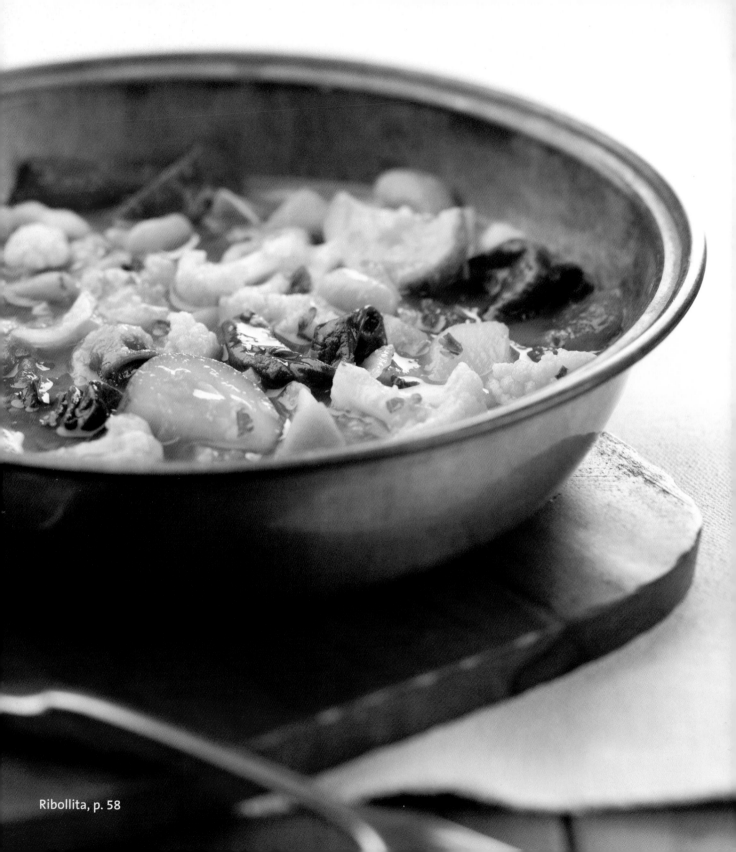

Ribollita, p. 58

CHAPTER 3
Soups and Stews

5-Minute Creamy Mushroom Soup | 44

Asopao de Pollo (Puerto Rican Chicken and Rice Soup) | 45

Baked Potato Soup | 46

Black Bean Soup with a Kick | 47

Butternut Squash Stew with Chickpeas | 48

Chickpea Soup with Orzo | 49

Cheddar Cheese and Broccoli Soup | 51

Creamy Tomato Soup | 52

Escarole and White Bean Soup | 53

Italian Minestrone | 54

Italian Sausage and White Bean Soup | 55

Oven Pork Stew with Sweet Potatoes and Shallots | 56

Ribollita | 58

Roasted Carrot Soup | 59

Tasty Tortilla Soup | 60

Wild Mushroom Soup | 61

5-Minute Creamy Mushroom Soup*

1/2 cup water

1/4 cup raw, unsalted cashews

2 tablespoons chopped onion

1–2 small garlic cloves

1/2 cup sliced button mushrooms

2 tablespoons chopped celery

2 teaspoons lemon juice

kosher salt, to taste

freshly ground black pepper, to taste

1 tablespoon chopped scallions (optional)

*Recipe courtesy of Andy Bellatti, RD

Cooking for one should still be satisfying and comforting. This exceptionally fast soup is ready in a jiffy. This soup has a delightful twist. A creamy texture imparted by heart-healthy cashews is used instead of butter or cream.

1 Add all ingredients to a blender or food processor until smooth.

2 Pour into a small saucepan and heat over medium-high heat for 3 minutes.

3 Lower the heat and simmer for 2 minutes. Top with scallions, if desired.

EXCHANGES/ CHOICES

1 Carbohydrate
1 High-Fat Meat
1 Fat

Calories **205**
  Calories from Fat **125**

Total Fat **14.0 g**
  Saturated Fat **2.5 g**
  Trans Fat **0.0 g**

Cholesterol **0 mg**

Sodium **25 mg**

Total Carbohydrate **15 g**
  Dietary Fiber **2 g**
  Sugars **4 g**

Protein **8 g**

Skim the Fat from Soups

Excess fat in a soup is not only unhealthy, but it makes the soup taste muddled and not fresh and clean. Here are three ways to de-fat a soup:

1. Chill the soup overnight in the refrigerator and then peel off and remove the fat that congeals with a large spoon.

2. Use a de-fatting pitcher, available at many cookware shops. This handy device helps separate the fat from the rest of the soup or stew liquid.

3. Prepare your soup or stew and then let it cool a bit at room temperature. Throw a layer of ice cubes on the top of the soup or stew. Wait a minute, then scoop the ice cubes off the surface. The excess fat should come along with it.

Asopao de Pollo*
(Puerto Rican Chicken and Rice Soup)

6 cups water

2 pounds boneless,
  skinless chicken breasts

1 tablespoon garlic powder

2 tablespoons olive oil

5 garlic cloves, very finely
  chopped

1 1/2 cups chopped onion

1 cup chopped green
  pepper

1/8 teaspoon freshly
  ground black pepper

1 tablespoon apple cider
  vinegar

2 8-ounce cans tomato
  sauce

2 small bay leaves

1/3 cup brown rice

1 cup peeled and sliced
  carrots

1/4 teaspoon hot red
  pepper flakes

My good friend Alex Oppenheimer's Puerto Rican heritage inspired this classic soup from the Caribbean. Alex taught me how to make this version, which is a nice twist from traditional American chicken soup.

1 In a large pot, bring the water to a boil. Meanwhile, trim any excess fat off the chicken and slice in half, for faster cooking. Season the chicken with garlic powder on all sides. In a large Dutch oven, heat the olive oil over medium-high heat. Add the chicken and brown on both sides for about 4 minutes per side. Remove the chicken from the pan and set aside.

2 Add the garlic and onion to the pan and sauté for 6–7 minutes. Add the green pepper and sauté for 3 minutes. Add in the black pepper, apple cider vinegar, tomato sauce, and bay leaves. Cover and bring to a simmer, stirring occasionally to prevent sticking.

3 Cut the chicken into bite-sized pieces and add to the pot and bring to a simmer.

4 Add the 6 cups of boiling water to the pot, stir and cover. Bring to a boil. Add the rice and carrots. Lower the heat and simmer, covered, for about 30–40 minutes. The rice should be tender and should split open. Remove the bay leaves before serving. Add in the red pepper flakes.

EXCHANGES/ CHOICES		
1/2 Starch	Calories **230**	Sodium **365 mg**
2 Vegetable	Calories from Fat **65**	Total Carbohydrate **15 g**
3 Lean Meat	Total Fat **7.0 g**	Dietary Fiber **3 g**
	Saturated Fat **1.3 g**	Sugars **5 g**
	Trans Fat **0.0 g**	Protein **26 g**
	Cholesterol **65 mg**	

*Recipe courtesy of
Alex Oppenheimer, RD

SERVES 6 SERVING SIZE 1 cup PREPARATION TIME 1 hour COOK TIME 1–1 1/2 hours

Baked Potato Soup

3 medium Idaho potatoes

3 slices lean turkey bacon

2 large onions, chopped

1/2 teaspoon salt

3 garlic cloves, minced

1 bay leaf

1/2 pound lean round steak, cubed into 1/2-inch pieces

3 1/2 cups 1% milk

1/2 teaspoon black pepper

1 1/2 cups chicken broth

3 scallions, chopped

3/4 cup reduced-fat finely shredded cheddar cheese

Love baked potatoes? Why not enjoy the roasted taste of potatoes in soup. All the elements of a comfort food in one warm bowl. Only use Idaho potatoes, also known as Russets; they produce the heartiest soup.

1 Preheat the oven to 400°F. Pierce each potato with a fork and bake the potatoes directly on the oven rack for 1–1 1/2 hours. Cool slightly. Scoop out the potatoes and mash. Discard the skins.

2 Cook the bacon in a large pot over medium heat until crisp. Remove bacon from the pan and crumble. Add the onions to the drippings and sauté for 5 minutes. Add the salt, garlic, and bay leaf and sauté for 2 minutes.

3 Add the steak and sauté for 5 minutes. Add the potato, milk, pepper, and broth and bring to a boil. Reduce the heat to simmer and cook for 10 minutes. Ladle the soup into bowls and top with sliced scallions, bacon, and cheese.

EXCHANGES/ CHOICES

1 Starch
1/2 Fat-Free Milk
2 Vegetable
1 Med-Fat Meat

Calories **260**
  Calories from Fat **65**
Total Fat **7.0 g**
  Saturated Fat **3.5 g**
  Trans Fat **0.0 g**
Cholesterol **45 mg**

Sodium **570 mg**
Total Carbohydrate **29 g**
  Dietary Fiber **2 g**
  Sugars **12 g**
Protein **21 g**

What Not to Freeze

Some soups and stews freeze great, but be careful not to freeze a soup or stew with these ingredients. Add them after you have defrosted the basic soup recipe.

Don't freeze soups with:
• potatoes
• yogurt
• eggs
• low-fat sour cream

Black Bean Soup with a Kick*

1 pound black beans,
  soaked in water and
  covered overnight

3 tablespoons olive oil

2 large white onions,
  chopped

1 cup diced red bell pepper

4 cloves garlic, minced

2 teaspoons chili powder

1 1/2 teaspoons ground
  cumin

1/2 teaspoon ground
  cayenne

1 1/2 teaspoons dried
  oregano

sea salt, to taste

freshly ground black
  pepper, to taste

3 cups low-fat, reduced-
  sodium chicken broth

1/4 cup lime juice

2 teaspoons brown sugar

GARNISH

1/2 cup plain nonfat Greek
  yogurt

1/2 cup minced cilantro

1 lime, cut into 8 thin slices

This is one of those slow-cooked soups that is worth every second of your time. This straightforward rich-flavored, black bean soup has a nice kick to it. I think that black bean soup truly is one of those must-have comfort soups.

1 Drain the soaked beans. Add the beans to a large Dutch oven and add fresh water to cover. Bring to a boil, lower the heat, partially cover the pot, and cook for 1 hour. Drain and rinse the beans and set aside.

2 Add the olive oil to a large saucepan over medium heat. Add the onion, red pepper, and garlic and sauté for about 6–7 minutes. Add the chili powder, cumin, cayenne, oregano, salt, and pepper and sauté for 1 minute.

3 Add the beans and broth and bring to a boil. Reduce the heat, partially cover the pan, and simmer on low heat for 2 hours. Remove 2 cups of the soup and purée it in a food processor or blender. Add back to the soup. Add in the lime juice and brown sugar. Heat for 1 minute.

4 Serve the soup in individual bowls with a dollop of yogurt, chopped cilantro, and a lime slice.

* Recipe courtesy of
Robin White

EXCHANGES/ CHOICES		
2 Starch	Calories **270**	Sodium **210 mg**
1 Vegetable	Calories from Fat **55**	Total Carbohydrate **41 g**
1 Lean Meat	Total Fat **6.0 g**	Dietary Fiber **13 g**
1/2 Fat	Saturated Fat **1.0 g**	Sugars **8 g**
	Trans Fat **0.0 g**	Protein **15 g**
	Cholesterol **0 mg**	

Butternut Squash Stew with Chickpeas

1 medium butternut
squash

2 teaspoons olive oil

1 large onion, chopped

3 garlic cloves, minced

1/2 pound small red
potatoes, unpeeled and
cut into quarters

1 cup low-fat, reduced-
sodium chicken broth

1 14-ounce can diced
tomatoes (try Fire
Roasted for more flavor),
undrained

3/4 teaspoon dried oregano

kosher salt, to taste

freshly ground black pepper,
to taste

1 15-ounce can chickpeas,
drained and rinsed

2 tablespoons reduced-fat,
natural creamy peanut
butter, stirred well until
smooth

2 tablespoons chopped
parsley

An unusual stew reminiscent of a traditional healthy African stew. By adding butternut squash to your diet, you add fiber and an abundance of vitamin A. Plus I've given you a pretty cool trick for cutting up this sometimes hard to handle winter squash. The flavors in this dish are hearty and will warm you up on a cool fall evening.

1   Prepare the butternut squash. Place the whole squash on the floor or rack of a microwave oven. Microwave the squash for 5 minutes. Carefully remove from the oven and let cool until it's cool enough to handle. With a sharp knife, cut the squash in half crosswise. Peel the skin off each half with the knife, cutting close to remove the skin only. Cut each half lengthwise. Remove the squash seeds from the bottom half of the squash and discard. Cut all the squash into 1-inch chunks. Set aside. This process makes cutting tough butternut squash easier as it helps loosen the skin.

2   Heat the oil in a large Dutch oven over medium heat. Add the onion and garlic and sauté for 5–6 minutes. Add the butternut squash and potatoes and stir to coat with the onions and garlic. Add the broth, tomatoes with juice, oregano, salt, and pepper. Bring to a boil. Lower the heat to a simmer, cover, and cook on medium-low heat for about 20 minutes, until squash and potatoes are tender. Some of the squash may become very soft.

3   Gently mix in the chickpeas and peanut butter and cook for 5 minutes. Garnish with chopped parsley.

EXCHANGES/ CHOICES		
1 1/2 Starch 1 Vegetable 1/2 Fat	Calories **160** Calories from Fat **30** Total Fat **3.5 g** Saturated Fat **0.5 g** Trans Fat **0.0 g** Cholesterol **0 mg**	Sodium **210 mg** Total Carbohydrate **28 g** Dietary Fiber **5 g** Sugars **6 g** Protein **6 g**

Chickpea Soup with Orzo

1 15-ounce can chickpeas, drained

1 medium onion, diced

2 garlic cloves, minced

6 cups low-fat, reduced-sodium chicken broth

1 1/2 cups fresh asparagus tips

4 ounces orzo (whole-wheat if you can find it)

kosher salt, to taste

freshly ground black pepper, to taste

GARNISH

strips of lemon zest from 1 lemon

2 tablespoons minced fresh parsley

This soup is a prime example of how the most basic ingredients can make a recipe so satisfying. It doesn't look like much when it's in the soup pot; however, the combination of creamy-textured pureed chickpeas and the burst of citrus flavor from the lemon, paired with the woodsy taste of fresh asparagus will find you making this humble soup often.

1 In a large saucepan, combine the chickpeas, onion, garlic, and broth and bring to a boil. Reduce the heat to low and simmer, uncovered, for about 20 minutes. Add more broth if the mixture becomes too thick.

2 Ladle about 1 cup of the chickpea mixture into a food processor or blender. Purée the mixture until smooth. Add back to the remaining soup in the pot. Add the asparagus, cover, and cook over low heat until asparagus is just tender.

3 Meanwhile, cook the orzo in a pot of lightly salted boiling water. Cook for about 8–9 minutes until tender. Drain and add to the soup. Season the soup with salt and pepper.

4 Ladle into bowls and top each serving with lemon zest and parsley.

EXCHANGES/ CHOICES		
1 1/2 Starch	Calories **170**	Sodium **590 mg**
1 Vegetable	Calories from Fat **15**	Total Carbohydrate **30 g**
1/2 Fat	Total Fat **1.5 g**	Dietary Fiber **5 g**
	Saturated Fat **0.2 g**	Sugars **6 g**
	Trans Fat **0.0 g**	Protein **10 g**
	Cholesterol **0 mg**	

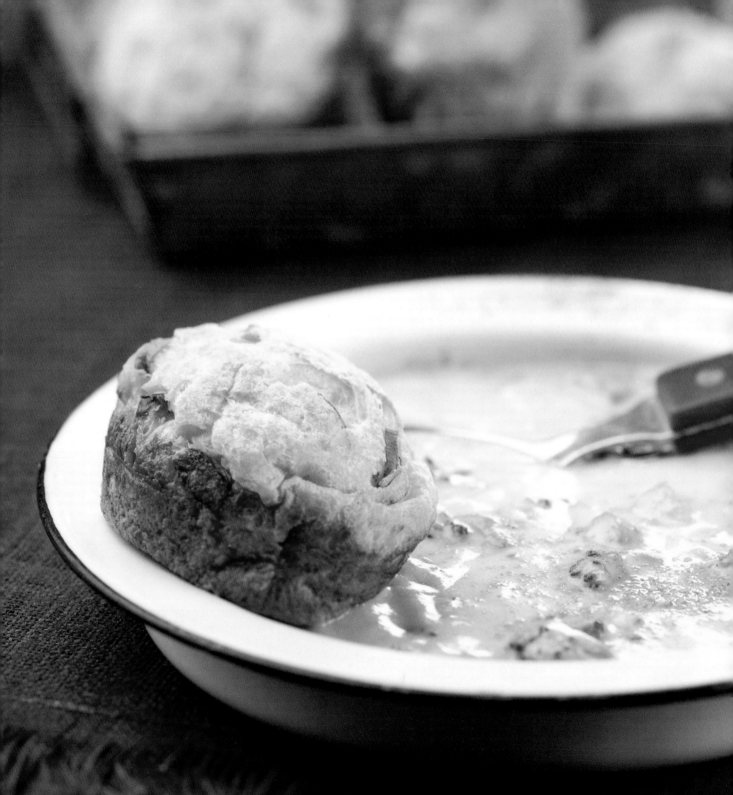

Cheddar Cheese and Broccoli Soup, p. 51; Parmesan Popovers, p. 30

Cheddar Cheese and Broccoli Soup

1 pound broccoli

1 tablespoon olive oil

1 onion, chopped

1 celery stalk, chopped

2 tablespoons all-purpose flour

1 14 1/2-ounce reduced-sodium chicken broth

1 12-ounce can evaporated fat-free milk

1 1/4 cups shredded, reduced-fat cheddar cheese (such as Cabot's 50% reduced-fat cheddar)

1/2 teaspoon freshly ground black pepper

1/4 teaspoon nutmeg

salt, to taste

The most satisfying comfort soup in my opinion is creamy and cheesy. As a kid, Cheddar Cheese and Broccoli Soup was always a staple in our kitchen; however, this version has been slimmed down considerably.

1 Trim and peel broccoli stems. Cut off 15 small florets. Coarsely chop enough remaining broccoli to equal 2 cups.

2 Blanch chopped broccoli and florets in boiling water just until bright green, about 2 minutes. Drain and set aside.

3 Heat olive oil in medium saucepan over medium heat. Sauté onion and celery until soft, about 5 minutes. Whisk in flour and cook 1 minute. Add broth and milk. Cook, stirring constantly, until mixture simmers and thickens, about 5 minutes.

4 Add chopped broccoli, cheese, pepper, nutmeg, and salt. Stir until cheese melts and soup is heated through, about 3 minutes. Garnish each bowl with reserved broccoli florets.

EXCHANGES/ CHOICES		
1 Fat-Free Milk 2 Vegetable 1 1/2 Fat	Calories **205** Calories from Fat **70**	Sodium **490 mg** Total Carbohydrate **20 g**
	Total Fat **8.0 g** Saturated Fat **3.5 g** Trans Fat **0.0 g**	Dietary Fiber **3 g** Sugars **12 g**
	Cholesterol **20 mg**	Protein **17 g**

Flavor Test

Here's how to season soups and stews like a professional chef and have a little fun in the kitchen. Take 3–4 small bowls or ramekins. Add 1/4 cup of the soup or stew you've prepared to each bowl. Add a different herb or spice you think might spike the flavor to each one. For example, if you are making a chicken soup, add fresh basil to one bowl, a little tarragon to another, dill to one, and thyme to another. Taste test with friends or family to see how each flavor changes or enhances the basic soup recipe. Pick a favorite and finish the soup recipe or let your guests add their favorite to their own bowl.

Creamy Tomato Soup*

1 tablespoon butter

3 cloves, minced garlic

1 tablespoon flour

1 1/2 cups fat-free half-and-half

1 14 1/2-ounce can crushed tomatoes with puree

1 14 1/2-ounce can reduced-fat, reduced-sodium chicken broth

1 teaspoon dried oregano

1 teaspoon dried basil

kosher salt, to taste

freshly ground black pepper, to taste

*Recipe courtesy of Molly Morgan, RD

I have always loved cream of tomato soup and this one is far and away better than the canned variety!

1 Heat the butter in a 3-quart saucepan over medium heat. Add the garlic and sauté for 1–2 minutes, keeping the garlic looking white.

2 Add in the flour and mix well. Add in the half and half and cook over medium heat until thickened and bubbly. Cook for an additional minute.

3 Add in the crushed tomatoes, broth, and spices. Bring to a boil, lower the heat, and simmer for 15 minutes. Season with salt and pepper.

EXCHANGES/ CHOICES		
1/2 Fat-Free Milk 2 Vegetable 1 Fat	Calories **130** Calories from Fat **40** Total Fat **4.5 g** Saturated Fat **2.6 g** Trans Fat **0.0 g** Cholesterol **10 mg**	Sodium **545 mg** Total Carbohydrate **17 g** Dietary Fiber **3 g** Sugars **8 g** Protein **6 g**

Simple Toppings

A simple garnish for soups or stews adds extra flavor, dimension, and beautiful presentation.

- Parmesan cheese (shredded or in shards—use a wide vegetable peeler to make long shards)
- Chopped chives
- Minced fresh herbs
- A swirl of Greek nonfat yogurt
- A few pieces of popcorn or crushed whole grain pretzels

Escarole and White Bean Soup

2 teaspoons olive oil

1 medium onion, chopped

2 garlic cloves, minced

1 large carrot, peeled and diced

1 celery stalk, diced

1 tablespoon flour

4 cups low-fat, reduced-sodium chicken broth

1 14-ounce can diced tomatoes, undrained

1 15-ounce can cannellini beans or other white beans, drained and rinsed

1 teaspoon dried oregano

1/2 teaspoon dried rosemary

2 cups washed and chopped escarole

2 tablespoons chopped fresh basil

1 1/2 teaspoon fresh lemon juice

kosher salt, to taste

freshly ground black pepper, to taste

This is one of my favorite soups—it's a terrific way to introduce super nutritious greens to your family. The escarole almost melts into the richly flavored broth.

1   Heat the olive oil in a large saucepot over medium heat. Add the onion, garlic, carrot, and celery and sauté for 6–8 minutes until softened. Add in the flour and cook while stirring. Cook for 1 minute.

2   Add in the broth, tomatoes, beans, oregano, and rosemary and bring to a boil. Lower the heat and simmer, uncovered, for 20 minutes.

3   Add in the escarole, and cook for 4 minutes until the escarole wilts. Add in the basil and cook for 1 minute. Add in the lemon juice, and season with salt and pepper.

EXCHANGES/ CHOICES		
1/2 Starch	Calories **110**	Sodium **495 mg**
2 Vegetable	Calories from Fat **20**	Total Carbohydrate **18 g**
1/2 Fat	Total Fat **2.0 g**	Dietary Fiber **5 g**
	Saturated Fat **0.3 g**	Sugars **4 g**
	Trans Fat **0.0 g**	Protein **6 g**
	Cholesterol **0 mg**	

Italian Minestrone

2 teaspoons olive oil

1/3 cup diced prosciutto

1 yellow onion, chopped

2 carrots, peeled and
coarsely chopped

2 garlic cloves, minced

1/2 small head green
cabbage, cored and
thinly sliced

1 14 1/2-ounce can diced
tomatoes, undrained

1 15-ounce can cannellini
beans, drained and
rinsed

5 cups low-fat, reduced-
sodium chicken broth

1 tablespoon freshly
chopped oregano

1 large zucchini, halved
and sliced into 1/2-inch
half moons

5 ounces shaped pasta

pinch cayenne pepper

sea salt, to taste

fresh ground black pepper,
to taste

1 tablespoon freshly
grated Parmesan cheese
per bowl

When Americans think of Italian soups, minestrone always comes to mind first. There are so many versions of this mélange of vegetables, tomatoes, and pasta, it's hard to make a culinary error when fixing it. Here's my version of the soup, streamlined to make it a bit easier than the versions I learned in Italy.

1 Heat the oil in a large saucepan over medium heat. Add the prosciutto and sauté for 2 minutes. Add the onions and carrots and sauté for 6–8 minutes. Add the garlic and sauté for 2 minutes.

2 Add in the cabbage, tomatoes, beans, and broth. Bring to a boil. Lower the heat and simmer, uncovered, for 20 minutes.

3 Add in the oregano, zucchini, and pasta. Raise the heat to medium and cook until the pasta is done, about 6–8 minutes. Season to taste with the sea salt, cayenne, and pepper. Sprinkle each bowl with Parmesan cheese.

EXCHANGES/ CHOICES		
1 Starch 1 Vegetable 1/2 Fat	Calories **120** Calories from Fat **25** Total Fat **3.0 g** Saturated Fat **1.2 g** Trans Fat **0.0 g** Cholesterol **5 mg**	Sodium **325 mg** Total Carbohydrate **17 g** Dietary Fiber **3 g** Sugars **4 g** Protein **7 g**

Italian Sausage and White Bean Soup

1 pound dried white beans (i.e., cannellini), soaked overnight

3 teaspoons olive oil, divided

2 garlic cloves, minced

3 carrots, diced

1/2 cup diced green pepper

1 medium onion, chopped

1 celery stalk, chopped

1 14 1/2-ounce can diced tomatoes, drained

3 cups low-fat, reduced-sodium chicken broth

2 cups water

1 large sprig fresh rosemary

1 pound low-fat, Italian turkey sausage, sliced

salt, to taste

pepper, to taste

3 tablespoons freshly grated Parmesan cheese

Another of my favorite recipes, this soup lets you have your sausage and eat it too! Filled with fiber and protein, this one is so delicious you'll forget that it's also really good for you. Make it for dinner and save a bowl for lunch the next day—it's even better when it sits overnight and the flavors meld together.

1   Drain the beans from their soaking water and set aside.

2   Heat 2 teaspoons of oil in a large Dutch oven or similar pan over medium heat. Add the garlic, carrots, green pepper, onion, and celery and sauté for about 10 minutes until soft, but not brown.

3   Add the beans, tomatoes, broth, water, and rosemary to the pot and bring to a boil. Reduce the heat and simmer for 1 to 1 1/2 hours until the beans are soft.

4   Heat the remaining oil in a large skillet over medium heat. Sear the sausage for about 4–5 minutes until lightly browned. Add the sausage to the pot and season with salt and pepper. Sprinkle with Parmesan cheese.

EXCHANGES/ CHOICES

2 Starch
1 Vegetable
3 Lean Meat

Calories **315**
  Calories from Fat **65**
Total Fat **7.0 g**
  Saturated Fat **1.6 g**
  Trans Fat **0.2 g**
Cholesterol **35 mg**

Sodium **525 mg**
Total Carbohydrate **40 g**
  Dietary Fiber **10 g**
  Sugars **6 g**
Protein **24 g**

Low-fat Croutons

Croutons make a great topping for a bowl of soup. Make your own. It's so easy!

1. Remove the crusts from bread and cut into cubes or shapes using a small cutter.

2. Place the breadcrumbs on a foil-lined broiler pan. Brush olive oil over the cubes. Broil until golden on both sides.

Oven Pork Stew with Sweet Potatoes and Shallots

1 tablespoon olive oil

1 pound boneless pork loin, cut into 1 1/2-inch pieces

1 medium onion, chopped

2 medium (5 ounces each) sweet potatoes, peeled and cut into 8 wedges

8 large shallots, peeled and left whole

4 garlic cloves, minced

3 tablespoons flour

1 2/3 cups fat-free, lower-sodium chicken broth

1/2 cup dry white wine (Pinot Grigio or Sauvignon Blanc)

1 tablespoon minced fresh thyme

kosher or sea salt, to taste

freshly ground black pepper, to taste

1/2 pound cremini or white button mushrooms, cleaned, stems removed, and cut in half

1/2 cup chopped fresh parsley

This dish is a beauty. The light purple color of the shallots contrasts nicely with the bright orange of the sweet potatoes. This is one of those classic stovetop-to-oven dishes that fills the kitchen with a heavenly aroma.

1 Preheat the oven to 350°F. Heat the olive oil in a large ovenproof Dutch oven or similar pan. Add the pork, in two batches, until the pork is well browned on all sides, about 6 minutes per batch. Remove the pork from the pan and set aside. Add in the onion, sweet potatoes, shallots, and garlic and sauté for 2–3 minutes.

2 Add the pork with any accumulated juices back into the pan and sprinkle with the flour. Cook for 1 minute, stirring continuously, until the flour is absorbed into the pork and vegetables. Add in the chicken broth, wine, thyme, salt, and pepper. Bring to a boil. Lower the heat and add in the mushrooms.

3 Transfer the pan to the oven and bake uncovered for 40–45 minutes or until the vegetables are tender. Sprinkle with parsley.

EXCHANGES/ CHOICES		
1 Starch	Calories **230**	Sodium **195 mg**
1 Vegetable	Calories from Fat **65**	Total Carbohydrate **22 g**
2 Lean Meat	Total Fat **7.0 g**	Dietary Fiber **3 g**
1 Fat	Saturated Fat **2.1 g**	Sugars **6 g**
	Trans Fat **0.0 g**	Protein **18 g**
	Cholesterol **40 mg**	

Oven Pork Stew with Sweet Potatoes and Shallots, p. 56

Ribollita

3 tablespoons olive oil

2/3 cup finely chopped red onion

1/2 cup finely chopped celery

1/2 cup finely chopped carrots

2 garlic cloves, minced

2 tablespoons minced parsley

1 32-ounce can tomatoes

1 medium potato, peeled and cut into 1-inch chunks

1 medium zucchini, halved, thinly sliced into 1/2-inch pieces

1/2 small head cauliflower, cut into bite-sized pieces

1 cup coarsely chopped green cabbage

1/2 cup chopped spinach

1 14-ounce can cannellini beans, drained

sea salt, to taste

freshly ground black pepper, to taste

water, to cover

1 1/2 cups day-old Italian bread, cut into 1/2-inch chunks

1 tablespoon olive oil

One of my all-time favorite soups hails from the Tuscany region of Italy where I have had bowlful after bowlful of this hearty soup/stew. Historically, the people of the region were so poor they used whatever they could find in the backyard garden plus some stale bread to concoct this winter soup that would fill their stomachs. The Tuscans' humble means are our gain!

1 Heat the olive oil in a large pot over medium-high heat. Add the red onion, celery, carrots, garlic, and parsley and sauté for 5–7 minutes until golden in color.

2 Add the tomatoes to a large bowl. With your hands, smash the tomatoes but leave some texture. Add the tomatoes, potato, zucchini, cauliflower, cabbage, spinach, beans, salt, pepper, and enough water to cover the entire mixture. Cook over medium-low heat for about 30 minutes. Add the bread and olive oil.

3 Place the soup back on the heat and cook over medium-low heat for 30 minutes.

4 Adjust and correct seasonings to taste.

EXCHANGES/ CHOICES		
1 Starch 2 Vegetable 1 1/2 Fat	Calories **190** Calories from Fat **70** Total Fat **8.0 g** Saturated Fat **1.1 g** Trans Fat **0.0 g** Cholesterol **0 mg**	Sodium **295 mg** Total Carbohydrate **26 g** Dietary Fiber **5 g** Sugars **6 g** Protein **6 g**

Roasted Carrot Soup*

1 pound carrots, cleaned and cut into 1-inch pieces

2 medium apples, peeled, cored, and cut into 16 wedges

1 small fennel bulb (white part only), cut into wedges

2 teaspoons olive oil

1 garlic clove, finely minced

1 tablespoon grated ginger

1/2 teaspoon kosher salt (optional)

3 1/2 cups low-fat, reduced-sodium chicken broth

2 tablespoons coarsely chopped dried cranberries

A creamy soup without the cream! Roasting carrots and apples brings out their natural highlights—sweetness and an earthy warmth. Fresh grated ginger further enhances the depth of flavor in this comforting fall soup.

1 Preheat oven to 400°F. Place carrots, apples, and fennel onto a baking sheet and drizzle with olive oil. Make sure to coat pieces evenly with oil. Bake in oven for 45–60 minutes. Carrots should be somewhat firm, but apples and fennel will be soft.

2 Remove carrots, apples, and fennel from oven with any accumulated juices and put into a large saucepan. Add garlic, ginger, and salt to saucepan. Pour chicken stock over vegetables. Bring to a boil and simmer for 15 minutes.

3 Transfer contents of saucepan to a blender, in batches, and puree until smooth. (Be very careful blending hot liquids.) Add more chicken broth to thin out soup to desired consistency.

4 Garnish each bowl with dried cranberries.

*Recipe courtesy of Pamela Braun

EXCHANGES/ CHOICES		
1/2 Fruit 3 Vegetable 1/2 Fat	Calories **130** Calories from Fat **25** Total Fat **3.0 g** Saturated Fat **0.4 g** Trans Fat **0.0 g** Cholesterol **0 mg**	Sodium **535 mg** Total Carbohydrate **25 g** Dietary Fiber **5 g** Sugars **15 g** Protein **4 g**

Tasty Tortilla Soup

2 teaspoons olive oil

1 small onion, chopped

2 garlic cloves, minced

2 teaspoons chili powder

4 cups low-fat, reduced-sodium chicken broth

1 14 1/2-ounce can diced tomatoes

1 medium zucchini, diced

1 yellow squash, diced

1 cup frozen yellow corn, thawed

3 corn tortillas

1/3 cup shredded reduced-fat cheddar cheese

In the time it would take to drive to your favorite Mexican restaurant, you can prepare this rich-tasting soup. The vegetables retain their bright color and firmer texture because they aren't cooked to death. The cheese melts very nicely so you get a bite of it in each spoonful.

1 Heat the oil in a large saucepan over medium heat. Add the onion and garlic and sauté for 5 minutes. Add the chili powder and sauté for 1 minute more.

2 Add the remaining ingredients except the tortillas and cheese. Bring to a boil, lower the heat, cover, and simmer for 25 minutes.

3 Meanwhile, cut the tortillas into 1/2-inch strips. Place the strips on a baking sheet. Bake the strips in a 350°F oven for about 5–6 minutes until the tortillas are lightly browned.

4 To serve, place some of the tortilla strips in a bowl. Pour soup over the tortillas. Top with a sprinkle of cheese.

EXCHANGES/CHOICES

1/2 Starch
1 Vegetable
1/2 Fat

Calories **85**
  Calories from Fat **20**
Total Fat **2.5 g**
  Saturated Fat **0.8 g**
  Trans Fat **0.0 g**
Cholesterol **0 mg**

Sodium **370 mg**
Total Carbohydrate **13 g**
  Dietary Fiber **2 g**
  Sugars **4 g**
Protein **5 g**

Herbal Ice Cubes

When you need to add flavor easily, just pop an herb ice cube into your stew or soup for instant flavor. You will most likely have fresh herbs left over from another recipe, so try this two-step method. Just add a cube and heat through your soup or stew.

1. Add a small sprig of herbs of your choice to an ice cube tray. Chop leafy herbs such as basil.

2. Add water to half fill the tray. The herbs will float to the top. Freeze, fill the tray with water, and freeze again.

Wild Mushroom Soup

2 tablespoons olive oil

4 garlic cloves, chopped

1 large onion, chopped

2 tablespoons fresh rosemary, minced

sea salt, to taste

freshly ground black pepper, to taste

1/4 pound fresh cremini mushrooms, cleaned and sliced

1/4 pound fresh shiitake mushrooms, cleaned and sliced

1/2 ounce dried porcini mushrooms

1/2 ounce dried chanterelle mushrooms

3 tablespoons brandy (optional)

1 small russet potato, diced into 1/2-inch pieces

1/4 cup half-and-half

6 cups low-fat, reduced-sodium chicken broth

4 tablespoons minced fresh parsley

This creamy, hearty soup awaits on the darkest days of winter. It's so rich and satisfying you'll swear you're cheating on your meal plan. Rather than thickening this soup with cream, a chopped russet potato is added to give the soup some heft, plus bonus fiber and vitamin C along the way.

1 Heat the olive oil in a large pot over medium heat. Add the garlic, onion, rosemary, salt, and pepper and cook for 3 minutes. Add in all of the mushrooms and cook for 5 minutes. Stir in the brandy, if using, and cook for 2 minutes.

2 Add in the half-and-half, chicken broth, and potato and bring to a boil. Reduce the heat and simmer, uncovered for 20 minutes.

3 Purée the soup in batches in a food processor or blender. Return the soup to the pot to reheat. Garnish each bowl with chopped parsley.

*Recipe courtesy of Pamela Braun

EXCHANGES/ CHOICES		
2 Vegetable 1 Fat	Calories **100** Calories from Fat **40** Total Fat **4.5 g** Saturated Fat **1.0 g** Trans Fat **0.0 g** Cholesterol **5 mg**	Sodium **390 mg** Total Carbohydrate **12 g** Dietary Fiber **2 g** Sugars **3 g** Protein **4 g**

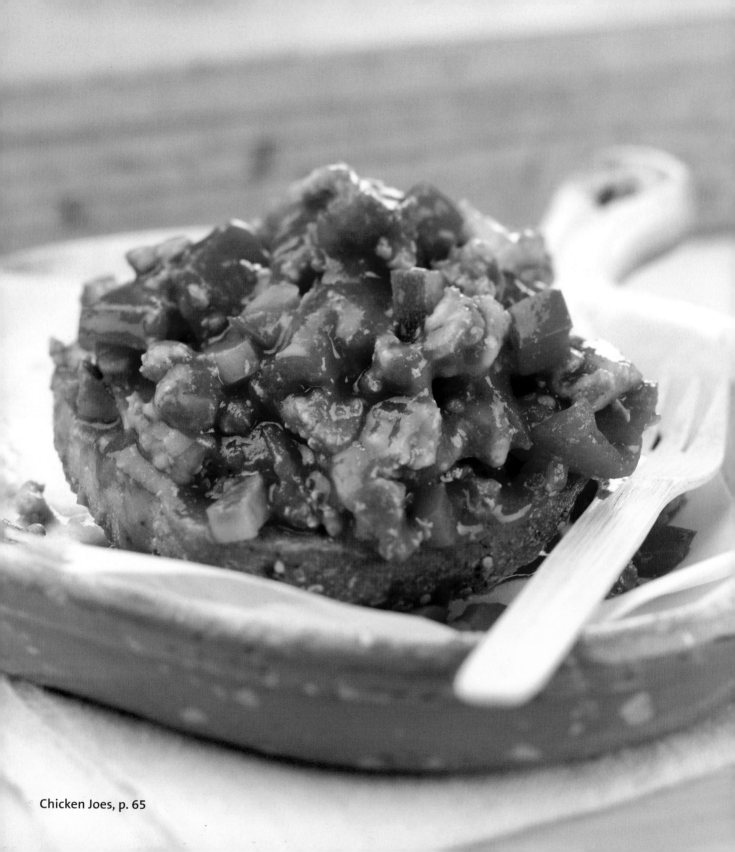

Chicken Joes, p. 65

CHAPTER 4
American Classics

BBQ Beef Sandwiches | 64

Chicken Joes | 65

Chicken Pot Pie with Phyllo | 66

Classic Free-Formed Meatloaf | 68

Classic Grilled Cheese | 69

Classic Mac 'n Cheese | 70

Everyday Taco Salad | 72

Filet Mignon with Spiced Pepper Crust | 73

Grilled Lamb Burgers | 74

Grilled Sirloin Salad | 75

Maple Glazed Pork Loin | 76

Orange Glazed Cornish Hens | 78

Oven Fried Cod | 79

Pan Grilled Beef with Mushroom Gravy | 80

Pepper Crushed Beef Tenderloin with Horseradish Sauce | 81

Roast Beef Hash | 82

Roast Beef Reubens | 83

Roast Chicken | 84

Spiced Beef Stew with Dried Fruits | 85

Slow Cooked BBQ Chicken | 86

Traditional Lump Crab Cakes | 89

Turkey Pesto Sandwiches | 90

Turkey Stroganoff | 91

BBQ Beef Sandwiches

1/2 cup low-sodium ketchup

1 tablespoon red wine vinegar

2 teaspoons brown sugar

1/2 teaspoon ground ginger

1/2 teaspoon chili powder

1/2 teaspoon Dijon mustard

1/2 teaspoon liquid smoke

8 ounces lean sirloin steak, trimmed of excess fat

4 small whole-wheat hamburger buns, split and toasted

One of my dear husband's favorite foods is a good old BBQ beef sandwich. I don't prepare a lot of beef dishes in my home, but when I can manipulate something he loves into something much lower in fat, salt, and sugar, I'm going to do it for him!

1   In a saucepan, combine the ketchup, vinegar, brown sugar, ginger, chili powder, mustard, and liquid smoke. Bring to a gentle boil, lower the heat, and simmer for 10 minutes.

2   Preheat an oven broiler or prepare an outdoor grill with the heat set to medium-high. Add the steak to a foil-lined broiler tray or set the steak on a well-oiled grilled rack. Brush one side of the steak with the BBQ sauce and broil or grill for about 5 minutes. Turn the steak over and brush on more of the sauce. Broil or grill an additional 4–5 minutes or until desired doneness. Reserve any remaining sauce for passing at the table.

3   Remove the steak from the broiler or grill to a carving board. Let the steak rest for 10 minutes. Thinly slice the steak on a bias. Place the steak on the bottom half of each bun. Top with the remaining bun half. Eat with a fork if necessary.

EXCHANGES/ CHOICES

2 Starch
2 Lean Meat

Calories **235**
  Calories from Fat **40**
Total Fat **4.5 g**
  Saturated Fat **1.2 g**
  Trans Fat **0.1 g**
Cholesterol **20 mg**

Sodium **255 mg**
Total Carbohydrate **35 g**
  Dietary Fiber **4 g**
  Sugars **14 g**
Protein **15 g**

Chicken Joes

3/4 pound ground chicken

1 small onion, minced

2 cloves garlic, minced

1 teaspoon chili powder

1/2 teaspoon paprika

salt, to taste

pepper, to taste

1 red or green pepper, chopped

3/4 cup diced zucchini

1 14 1/2-ounce can diced tomatoes, drained

1/2 cup bottled BBQ sauce (look for a brand with the lowest amount of sugar)

4 toasted whole-wheat hamburger buns

OK, so time for a confession. While we always had home-cooked meals, we also always had a can of Sloppy Joe mix tucked into the corner of the pantry for when we got lazy. Knowing now that processed foods are not healthy, I developed these Chicken Joes with all the same taste of the Sloppy Joes of childhood. With extra vegetables, this version makes the grade.

1 In a large skillet, cook the ground chicken, onion, garlic, chili powder, paprika, salt, and pepper over medium heat until meat is browned, about 5–6 minutes.

2 Add in the green or red pepper and zucchini and cook over low heat for about 5 minutes, until vegetables are tender. Add the diced tomatoes and BBQ sauce and simmer for 10 minutes.

3 Serve the mixture over half of a toasted bun.

EXCHANGES/ CHOICES	Calories **145** Calories from Fat **40**	Sodium **340 mg** Total Carbohydrate **17 g**
1 Starch 1 Med-Fat Meat	Total Fat **4.5 g** Saturated Fat **1.2 g** Trans Fat **0.0 g**	Dietary Fiber **3 g** Sugars **6 g**
	Cholesterol **30 mg**	Protein **10 g**

Chicken Pot Pie with Phyllo

1 pound boneless skinless chicken breasts, diced into 1/2-inch pieces

1 1/2 teaspoon garlic powder

freshly ground black pepper, to taste

2 cups fat-free, reduced-sodium chicken broth

1/2 cup water

1 teaspoon olive oil

10 ounces cremini mushrooms, cut into 1/2-inch pieces (about 3 cups)

1 garlic clove, finely chopped

kosher or sea salt, to taste

1 pound small red potatoes, unpeeled and cut into quarters

5 sprigs fresh thyme

3 medium (1 cup total) carrots, diced into 1/2-inch pieces

1 large (2 cups total) onion, diced

1 1/2 cups 1% milk

1/2 cup half-and-half

6 tablespoons flour

8 ounces frozen peas

1/2 cup minced flat leaf parsley

8 sheets (9 × 14-inch) phyllo dough

butter-flavored spray

There is nothing more comforting than chicken and veggies in a lusciously thick sauce topped with a flaky crust. The earthy aroma of this dish will fill your kitchen and call everyone to dinner. The secret to this ultimate comfort food? By using butter-flavored spray and phyllo dough we slash all the saturated fat and calories found in a typical pie crust topping. The phyllo dough topping is infinitely more interesting than a standard crust.

1   Preheat the oven to 400°F. Season the diced chicken with garlic powder and freshly ground pepper and set aside. In a 2-quart saucepan, bring the chicken stock and water to a boil.

2   Meanwhile, heat the olive oil in a medium skillet and add the mushrooms and garlic. Season lightly with salt and pepper. Cook for 5 minutes or until mushrooms are soft. Once the mushrooms soften, set them aside in a bowl. Strain any liquid from the mushrooms.

3   Add in the potatoes and thyme leaves and lower the heat to medium. Simmer the potatoes for about 8 minutes until tender. With a slotted spoon, remove the potatoes and thyme to a bowl. Discard the thyme leaves. Add the carrots and onions to the stock and simmer for 4 minutes. With a slotted spoon remove the carrots and onions to the same bowl with the potatoes.

4   Add the chicken to the stock and simmer the chicken for 3 minutes. With a slotted spoon, remove the chicken to

EXCHANGES/ CHOICES	Calories **180**	Sodium **180 mg**
1 1/2 Starch	Calories from Fat **20**	Total Carbohydrate **26 g**
1 Vegetable	Total Fat **2.5 g**	Dietary Fiber **3 g**
1 Lean Meat	Saturated Fat **0.9 g**	Sugars **5 g**
	Trans Fat **0.0 g**	Protein **13 g**
	Cholesterol **25 mg**	

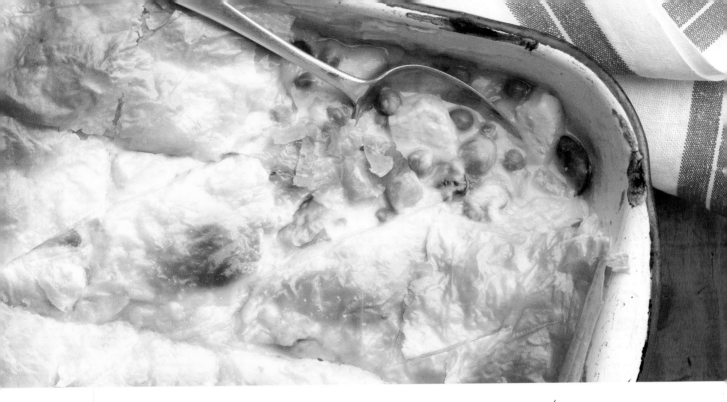

the same bowl with the vegetables. Reduce the stock until reduced to 1/2 cup, about 10 minutes.

5 Meanwhile, whisk the milk, half-and-half, and flour together in a bowl until very smooth. When the stock is reduced, slowly add the milk mixture to the stock, constantly stirring until thickened, but smooth. Add the sauce to the vegetables and season with salt and pepper. Add in the reserved mushrooms, peas, and parsley, and mix well.

6 Pour the mixture into a 9 × 13-inch pan. Set aside.

7 Spread one sheet of phyllo out onto a very lightly floured surface. Be sure to cover the remaining sheets of phyllo with a towel to avoid exposing to air. The phyllo will crack if exposed. Coat with the butter spray. Add another sheet of phyllo on top of the first sheet and coat with spray. Repeat this process until all 8 sheets are used.

8 Carefully lift the phyllo dough stack and place over the chicken vegetable filling. Tuck the edges under. With a sharp knife, make 3 diagonal slashes across the top of the dough. This will allow steam to escape.

9 Bake the chicken pot pie, uncovered, for about 30 minutes until the top is puffed and golden brown. Remove from the oven and let stand for about 5 minutes. Cut into squares.

Classic Free-Formed Meatloaf

cooking spray

1 1/2 teaspoons olive oil

1 cup finely chopped onion

2 garlic cloves, minced

3/4 pound 93–98% extra lean ground beef

3/4 pound ground lean pork

3/4 pound ground veal

1/2 cup tomato ketchup

1 tablespoon Dijon mustard

1 1/2 teaspoons Worcestershire sauce

3/4 cup fresh breadcrumbs (preferably made from Italian bread)

1 egg

1/2 cup finely minced parsley

kosher salt, to taste

freshly ground black pepper, to taste

By combining three different ground meats, this classic meatloaf stays extra moist. Baking without a pan ensures that the sides will be crusty and full of flavor, a texture that is far more appealing than meatloaf that tastes steamed when put into a loaf pan. This free-formed meatloaf is sure to be a family favorite.

1 Preheat the oven to 350°F. Coat a large baking sheet with cooking spray and set aside.

2 Heat the olive oil in a large skillet over medium heat. Add the onion and sauté for 4 minutes. Add in the garlic and sauté for 1 minute. Add the onions and garlic to a large mixing bowl.

3 Add the remaining ingredients to the bowl and mix well with your hands, but don't over handle the meat. The mixture should just be combined.

4 Turn the meat mixture onto the prepared baking sheet. Form the mixture into a large oval loaf.

5 Bake the meatloaf for 50 minutes to 1 hour until the internal temperature reaches 160. The meatloaf should be nicely browned and the edges should look crusty. If desired, broil the meatloaf for a few minutes to enhance the color.

6 Remove the meatloaf from the oven and let rest for 15 minutes before slicing.

EXCHANGES/ CHOICES		
1/2 Carbohydrate 2 Lean Meat	Calories **130** Calories from Fat **35** Total Fat **4.0 g** Saturated Fat **1.4 g** Trans Fat **0.0 g** Cholesterol **65 mg**	Sodium **210 mg** Total Carbohydrate **6 g** Dietary Fiber **0 g** Sugars **3 g** Protein **16 g**

Classic Grilled Cheese

BASIC SANDWICH

cooking spray (original or butter flavored)

2 slices whole-wheat bread (regular or light wheat)

2 ounces lower-fat cheese (such as Cabot's 75% reduced-fat cheddar)

OPTIONAL TOPPINGS
(pick one or a combination)

1 teaspoon sundried tomato, minced

1 tablespoon goat cheese (if using, only use 1 slice regular cheese in the basic sandwich)

jalapeño peppers, to taste

1 ounce (1 slice) prosciutto or any other ham

sliced tomato

I polled my family and friends by asking, "What is your favorite comfort food?" The unanimous answer was grilled cheese, so I had to include it here. Along with the basic recipe, I've added a few special toppings so that you can turn this classic sandwich into something memorable. Add Creamy Tomato Soup (page 52), share with a friend, and enter comfort food heaven!

1 Assemble sandwich with 2 slices of cheese and selected toppings, if any.

2 Preheat a nonstick pan on medium-low heat for 30 seconds. Spray the bottom of the pan with cooking spray and toast the sandwich on one side for 2–3 minutes until the bread is browned. Press down on the sandwich occasionally with a spatula.

3 Flip the sandwich, and toast for another 2–3 minutes until the second side is browned and the cheese is adequately melted.

4 Cut sandwich in half and serve immediately.

EXCHANGES/ CHOICES		
1 Starch	Calories **130**	Sodium **330 mg**
1 Lean Meat	Calories from Fat 30	Total Carbohydrate **12 g**
	Total Fat **3.5 g**	Dietary Fiber **2 g**
	Saturated Fat **1.7 g**	Sugars **2 g**
	Trans Fat **0.0 g**	Protein **13 g**
	Cholesterol **10 mg**	

Cheesy!

Cheese is synonymous with comfort food, but it's not always as easy to cook with as it is to eat cold. Here are some tips for creamy, smooth cheese.

• Cheese is a high protein food. When exposed to too much heat, the protein bonds break and will form curds or clumps. Many cheeses will only tolerate brief gentle heat.

• The residual heat in freshly cooked pasta, soup, or scrambled eggs is usually enough to melt cheese smoothly.

• If your cheese gets stringy when stirred into soups or sauces add a bit of something acidic—wine or lemon juice—to the cheese before melting it.

Classic Mac 'n' Cheese

2 3/4 cups 1% milk, divided

1/4 cup half-and-half

1/2 large onion, peeled and thinly sliced

1 bay leaf

5 whole peppercorns

12 ounces elbow macaroni

3 tablespoons cornstarch

1/2 teaspoon dry mustard

1 1/2 cups finely shredded reduced-fat extra sharp cheddar cheese (white or yellow)

1 tablespoon freshly grated Parmesan cheese

1 teaspoon salt

1/2 teaspoon fresh ground black pepper

TOPPING

3/4 cup fresh breadcrumbs (preferably made from Italian bread, but whole-wheat bread is fine)

2 teaspoons olive oil

You wouldn't believe it but this Mac 'n' Cheese has no butter in it at all. By infusing the milk with an onion, bay leaf, and peppercorns, the sauce has wonderful flavor, so there's no need for added fat. This Mac 'n' Cheese will be a hit with kids and adults, too. For a classic look use yellow cheddar; for a more sophisticated style use white cheddar.

1   Preheat the oven to 375°F. Coat an 8 × 8-inch square baking pan with cooking spray.

2   In a heavy bottomed 2-quart saucepan, combine 2 cups milk, half-and-half, onion, bay leaf, and peppercorns. Bring to a light boil, lower the heat, and simmer on medium-low heat for 20 minutes to allow the onion and spices to infuse into the milk. Using a strainer, strain the infused milk from the onion and spices and return the strained milk to the saucepan.

3   While the milk is simmering, bring a pot of salted water to a boil. Add the elbow macaroni and cook for 4–5 minutes. (This is less time than the package directions. You want the macaroni undercooked. This prevents the pasta from becoming too mushy in the casserole.) Drain, add to a large bowl, and set aside.

4   In a medium bowl, mix the remaining 3/4 cup of milk with the cornstarch. Whisk until well combined. Add half the milk mixture in the saucepan to the milk cornstarch mixture in the bowl and whisk for 1 minute. Add the milk cornstarch mixture back into the saucepan.

EXCHANGES/ CHOICES	Calories **185**	Sodium **300 mg**
	Calories from Fat **40**	Total Carbohydrate **26 g**
2 Starch	Total Fat **4.5 g**	Dietary Fiber **1 g**
1 Lean Meat	Saturated Fat **2.3 g**	Sugars **3 g**
	Trans Fat **0.0 g**	Protein **10 g**
	Cholesterol **10 mg**	

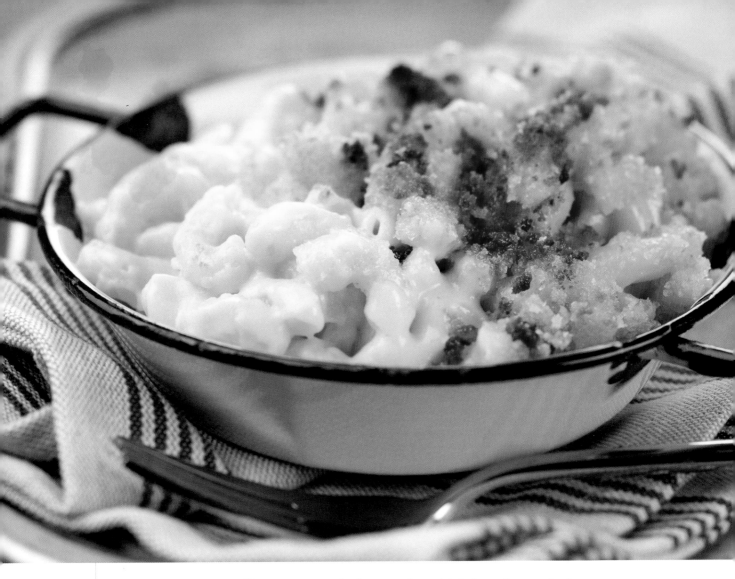

Bring the entire milk mixture to a boil on medium-high heat. Lower the heat to medium and cook until thickened, about 5–7 minutes. Mixture will still be on the thin side. Reduce the heat to low and simmer for 4–5 minutes.

5 Remove the pot from the stove. Whisk in the dry mustard, cheeses, salt, and pepper. Add the cheese sauce to the pasta and mix well. The mixture should look soupy.

6 Pour the macaroni and cheese mixture into the prepared pan. Combine the fresh breadcrumbs and olive oil in a small bowl and mix well. Sprinkle the top of the macaroni and cheese with the bread topping. Bake for 20–25 minutes until topping is light brown and macaroni and cheese is bubbly.

Everyday Taco Salad

2 teaspoons olive oil

1 pound 95–96% lean beef

1/2 cup minced onions

1 tablespoon chili powder

1/2 teaspoon ground cumin

1/2 teaspoon ground coriander

1/4 cup commercially prepared hot or mild salsa

6 cups shredded lettuce

2 small tomatoes, diced

1/2 large avocado, diced

36 baked tortilla chips

Don't even think about stopping off at a fast food restaurant when you want a taco salad. Make it yourself. Although taco salad may seem more Mexican than American, I include it here in American Classics because it's a quick, easy meal that's become popular in the U.S.

1 Heat the olive oil in a large skillet over medium-high heat. Add the beef and onions and sauté for 2 minutes. Add in the chili powder, cumin, and coriander and sauté until beef is cooked through. Drain any excess fat. Add in the salsa.

2 For each serving, top 3/4 cup of the lettuce with some of the meat mixture, tomatoes, avocado, and tortilla chips.

EXCHANGES/ CHOICES		
1/2 Starch	Calories **155**	Sodium **160 mg**
1 Vegetable	Calories from Fat **65**	Total Carbohydrate **10 g**
1 Lean Meat	Total Fat **7.0 g**	Dietary Fiber **3 g**
1 Fat	Saturated Fat **1.8 g**	Sugars **2 g**
	Trans Fat **0.1 g**	Protein **13 g**
	Cholesterol **35 mg**	

Filet Mignon with Spiced Pepper Crust

1 tablespoon cracked black pepper

1/2 teaspoon garlic powder

1/8 teaspoon kosher salt

2 teaspoons brandy

4 (4 ounces each) filet mignons, trimmed of fat

high heat canola oil cooking spray

This is how to cook a piece of beef: In its simplest form, unadorned, and with flavor in every bite. Pan searing is one of the best ways to control the cooking time on the beef. It's the way I teach beginner cooks how to get meat right every time. Just purchase the best quality beef you can afford and this steak is nothing less than spectacular.

1   Combine the pepper, garlic powder, salt, and brandy. Rub on one side of each filet.

2   Coat a large skillet (preferably cast iron) with high heat canola oil cooking spray. Heat the skillet to high heat. Add the filets, pepper mixture side down. Sprinkle the remaining pepper mixture over the other side of the filets. Sear the filets on one side for about 6–7 minutes. Turn the steaks over and continue searing about 5 minutes, turning down the heat to medium high, if necessary. Cook the steaks according to your preference.

EXCHANGES/ CHOICES	Calories **150**	Sodium **105 mg**
	Calories from Fat **55**	Total Carbohydrate **1 g**
3 Lean Meat	Total Fat **6.0 g**	Dietary Fiber **1 g**
	Saturated Fat **2.2 g**	Sugars **0 g**
	Trans Fat **0.0 g**	Protein **21 g**
	Cholesterol **60 mg**	

Grilled Lamb Burgers

1 pound lean ground lamb

1/2 cup minced cilantro

2 tablespoons minced red onion

2 tablespoons fat-free feta cheese

1/2 teaspoon cumin

1/4 teaspoon coriander

1/4 teaspoon cayenne pepper

1/4 teaspoon salt

1/4 teaspoon fresh ground black pepper

I had to do a burger for American classics, but I decided to try lamb burgers instead of a traditional beef burger. With a few exotic spices, this might start a new trend in burgers. As a matter of fact, I have seen more and more trendy restaurants serve lamb burgers, so I guess I am not too far off the mark!

1   In a medium bowl, mix together all ingredients, just until combined. (Avoid over handling the meat.) Gently form into 4 patties.

2   Grill or broil the patties 6 inches from the heat source for about 4–5 minutes per side.

3   Serve on a toasted bun with lettuce and tomato, if desired.

EXCHANGES/ CHOICES		
4 Lean Meat	Calories **180**	Sodium **355 mg**
	Calories from Fat **65**	Total Carbohydrate **2 g**
	Total Fat **7.0 g**	Dietary Fiber **0 g**
	Saturated Fat **3.0 g**	Sugars **1 g**
	Trans Fat **0.0 g**	Protein **26 g**
	Cholesterol **85 mg**	

Grilled Sirloin Salad

RUB

1 tablespoon chili powder

2 teaspoons dried oregano

1 teaspoon dried thyme

1/2 teaspoon garlic powder

1/2 teaspoon onion powder

1/2 teaspoon salt

1/4 teaspoon fresh ground black pepper

1 pound boneless beef top sirloin steak

SALAD

1 cup frozen yellow corn, thawed

1 red pepper, sliced into thin strips

1/2 red onion, thinly sliced

1 tablespoon minced parsley

2 tablespoons olive oil

1 tablespoon red wine vinegar

1 teaspoon fresh lemon juice

4 cups salad greens

1/4 cup crumbled blue cheese (optional)

Comfort food is not just limited to cold wintry nights. In the summer, the smokiness of this beef cooking on the outdoor grill might mean you have to comfort all the neighbors!

1   Combine the rub ingredients and spread over both sides of the steak. Place the steak over medium-high heat of a grill and grill for 9–12 minutes or longer to your liking.

2   Meanwhile, combine the corn, red pepper, red onion, and parsley. Add in the oil, vinegar, and lemon juice. Mix well.

3   Remove steak from grill and thinly slice on a bias.

4   For each serving, place salad greens on plate, top with corn mixture and slices of beef. Garnish with blue cheese.

EXCHANGES/ CHOICES		
1/2 Starch	Calories **255**	Sodium **355 mg**
1 Vegetable	Calories from Fat **100**	Total Carbohydrate **14 g**
3 Lean Meat	Total Fat **11.0 g**	Dietary Fiber **4 g**
1 Fat	Saturated Fat **2.2 g**	Sugars **4 g**
	Trans Fat **0.0 g**	Protein **26 g**
	Cholesterol **60 mg**	

Maple Glazed Pork Loin

SAUCE

1/3 cup fresh orange juice

4 tablespoons pure maple syrup

1 tablespoon coarse-ground Dijon mustard

2 teaspoons reduced-sodium soy sauce

1 teaspoon dark brown sugar

1/2 teaspoon ground cinnamon

PORK

3 tablespoons all-purpose flour

1 tablespoon granulated sugar

1/2 teaspoon kosher salt

1/4 teaspoon freshly ground black pepper

1 tablespoon canola oil

2 (1 pound each) lean pork tenderloins, patted dry

With a minimum amount of time and only a few ingredients from your pantry, turn an American favorite, pork tenderloin, into one that rivals the version from your favorite Asian restaurant.

1 Preheat oven to 400°F. Add a rack large enough to accommodate the pork tenderloins in a large baking pan. Coat the rack with cooking spray.

2 Whisk together all the sauce ingredients in a small bowl and set aside.

3 Mix together the flour, sugar, salt, and pepper. Spread the mixture onto a large baking sheet. Roll each pork tenderloin in the flour mixture. Shake off the excess. You will have about 1 1/2 tablespoons of flour mixture left over to discard. Pork should just be lightly coated. Do not do this in advance, as the flour will become gummy and pasty.

4 Heat the oil in a 12-inch skillet (preferably stainless steel or cast iron) over medium-high heat until there are light wisps of smoke. Add the pork tenderloins to the pan, leaving room in between each one. Curl the pork tenderloins if necessary to fit them in the pan.

5 Sear the pork for about 4 minutes per side until nicely browned. Add the pork tenderloins side-by-side to the prepared baking pan and set aside.

EXCHANGES/ CHOICES		
1/2 Carbohydrate 3 Lean Meat	Calories **160** Calories from Fat **40**	Sodium **205 mg** Total Carbohydrate **10 g**
	Total Fat **4.5 g** Saturated Fat **1.0 g** Trans Fat **0.0 g** Cholesterol **55 mg**	Dietary Fiber **0 g** Sugars **8 g** Protein **20 g**

6 Add the sauce to the pan and lower the heat to medium. Reduce the sauce to half its volume, scraping up any accumulated browned bits, about 5 minutes. The sauce should be a light mahogany color.

7 Brush 1/3 of the glaze over the pork tenderloins. Roast for about 20 minutes. Add another 1/3 of the glaze and continue to roast for 10 minutes. Add the remaining glaze and roast for 5 minutes.

8 Remove the pork from the oven, tent with foil, and let rest for 15 minutes before slicing.

How to Sauté the Right Way

American cooking often includes simple sautéing. Many of my students lament that their foods come out watery or flat-tasting after what they thought was sautéing. Here's how to have tasty, beautiful sautéed foods:

MAKE SURE THE FOOD YOU SAUTÉ IS VERY DRY.

Before putting the food into the pan, pat the surface of the food with paper towels to absorb excess moisture. If you don't, excess moisture will cause your food to steam rather than sauté.

JACK UP THE HEAT.

A good sauté calls for lots of heat. Put the food in the pan only when the pan and any oil you add is hot. Monitor the heat, so you don't burn anything, but don't turn it too low.

LEAVE LOTS OF ROOM IN BETWEEN THE FOODS YOU ARE SAUTÉING.

Don't crowd chicken pieces and mushrooms in one layer. When foods are piled high on top of each other, it creates steam, and food will not brown up nicely.

DON'T FLIP CONSTANTLY.

Let the food rest on the heat in one spot so it will properly brown. Then, flip it. Resist the urge to poke and prod food too much.

Orange Glazed Cornish Hens*

1 tea bag (e.g., Earl Grey)

2 medium oranges

1/2 cup no-sugar-added orange marmalade

4 (1 pound each) Rock Cornish hens, thawed if frozen

1/2 teaspoon pepper

salt, to taste

2 medium onions, sliced

8 sprigs fresh rosemary

8 sprigs fresh thyme

Cornish hens are a forgotten bird. I like to cook with them because their meat is hearty, but they are small, so it's easy to exercise portion control. This recipe is festive enough for holiday time and easy enough for jazzing up everyday dinners.

1 Preheat oven to 375°F. Fit a roasting pan with rack. In a small saucepan, steep tea bag in 1/4 cup boiling water for 5 minutes. Discard tea bag. Squeeze juice from 1 orange into tea, and stir in marmalade until melted. Keep warm. Cut remaining orange into quarters (do not peel).

2 Remove and discard giblets from hens. Wash and dry hens thoroughly and sprinkle cavities with pepper and salt. Loosen breast skin slightly. Stuff large cavity of each hen with 1 orange quarter, 1/4 of the onion slices, 1 rosemary sprig, and 1 thyme sprig. Tie legs together with kitchen string. Place hens, breast-side up, on rack in roasting pan. Brush hens (over and under skin) with about one-fourth of glaze. Pour enough water into pan to cover bottom (water should not reach rack).

3 Roast hens on middle oven rack, basting over and under skin every 20 minutes with remaining glaze, until hens are browned and juices run clear, about 1 hour. Let hens stand 10 minutes. Discard rosemary, thyme, onions, and orange from cavities of hens. Garnish with remaining rosemary and thyme sprigs. Discard skin before eating.

*Adapted from *Eat To Beat Diabetes* (Readers Digest, 2007)

EXCHANGES/ CHOICES		
3 Lean Meat	Calories **140**	Sodium **60 mg**
	Calories from Fat **30**	Total Carbohydrate **3 g**
	Total Fat **3.5 g**	Dietary Fiber **0 g**
	Saturated Fat **1.0 g**	Sugars **2 g**
	Trans Fat **0.0 g**	Protein **22 g**
	Cholesterol **100 mg**	

Oven Fried Cod

1/4 cup plus 2 tablespoons all-purpose flour, divided

salt, to taste

pepper, to taste

2 eggs

1 tablespoon reduced-fat mayonnaise

pinch cayenne pepper

3/4 cup panko breadcrumbs (look for panko breadcrumbs in the Asian section of your grocery store)

2 tablespoons finely minced fresh parsley

4 (4 ounces each) cod filets, 1 1/2 inches thick (halibut or haddock also work well)

I like to serve this oven fried fish with the Rustic Garlic and Olive Oil Mashed Potatoes (see page 32). The cod is simply prepared and is great for the next day's lunch served on a whole-wheat bun with lettuce and tomato. Yes, you can have fried fish, and this version has the familiar crunch that everyone craves!

1   Preheat the oven to 425°F. Coat a wire rack with cooking spray. Set the wire rack on a baking sheet lined with foil. Set aside.

2   Place 1/4 cup of the flour, salt, and pepper on a large plate. Whisk the eggs, the remaining 2 tablespoons of flour, mayonnaise, and cayenne pepper in a bowl. Whisk until the flour and mayonnaise are fully incorporated and there are no lumps.

3   Mix together the breadcrumbs and parsley and place on a second large plate.

4   Coat the cod lightly with the flour, shaking off any excess. Dip the floured cod in the beaten egg mixture. Finally, roll the cod in the breadcrumbs.

5   Place all the cod filets evenly spaced on the prepared rack and bake for about 25 minutes until the fish is cooked through and the crust is golden brown.

EXCHANGES/ CHOICES		
1 Starch 3 Lean Meat	Calories **225** Calories from Fat **40** Total Fat **4.5 g** Saturated Fat **1.2 g** Trans Fat **0.0 g** Cholesterol **155 mg**	Sodium **150 mg** Total Carbohydrate **19 g** Dietary Fiber **1 g** Sugars **1 g** Protein **26 g**

Pan Grilled Beef with Mushroom Gravy

2 (8 ounces each) lean beef tenderloin steaks (about 1/3-inch thick)

kosher salt, to taste

freshly ground black pepper, to taste

2 teaspoons canola oil

2 garlic cloves, minced

1/2 cup minced onions

1 cup sliced cremini mushrooms

1/2 cup low-fat, reduced-sodium beef stock

1/3 cup fat-free sour cream

2 teaspoons Dijon mustard

2 tablespoons minced parsley

Back in the 1960s, a dish like this was pretty standard in our house. Easy to prepare, but dreadfully high in fat in calories. Today, I have learned how to slim down this classic favorite. It's still very similar to the original, but you can have this dish more often.

1   Cut beef tenderloin steaks in half, to have a total of 4 steaks. Season with salt and pepper. Bring to room temperature about 30 minutes prior to cooking.

2   Heat the oil in a large skillet over medium-high heat until almost smoking. Sear the steaks for 2–3 minutes on each side to form a nice crust. Remove steaks from the skillet and keep warm.

3   Add the garlic and onions to the skillet and sauté for 3 minutes. Add the mushrooms and sauté for 3 minutes until mushrooms just begin to release their moisture. Stir in the stock, bring to a boil, cover, and simmer on medium-low heat until mushrooms are soft, about 3 minutes. Remove the skillet from the heat and whisk in the sour cream and mustard.

4   Serve the steaks with the mushroom gravy. Garnish with minced parsley.

EXCHANGES/ CHOICES	Calories **200**	Sodium **185 mg**
	Calories from Fat **70**	Total Carbohydrate **7 g**
1/2 Carbohydrate	Total Fat **8.0 g**	Dietary Fiber **1 g**
3 Lean Meat	Saturated Fat **2.5 g**	Sugars **2 g**
1/2 Fat	Trans Fat **0.0 g**	Protein **2 g**
	Cholesterol **60 mg**	

Pepper Crushed Beef Tenderloin with Horseradish Sauce

1 2-pound beef tenderloin

2 teaspoons olive oil

4 tablespoons dry breadcrumbs

3 tablespoons finely minced parsley

2 garlic cloves, minced to paste

1 1/2 teaspoons coarsely ground black pepper

1/2 teaspoon kosher salt

SAUCE

1 cup fat-free sour cream

3 tablespoons prepared horseradish

1 teaspoon grated lemon zest

1/2 teaspoon Worcestershire sauce

1/4 teaspoon hot sauce

salt, to taste

This recipe is a showstopper! Breadcrumbs, garlic, and parsley enhance the juicy tenderloin's flavor. The horseradish and sour cream sauce has a cool spiciness. Serve the leftovers cold for great lunch sandwiches. When you need to impress, this is your winning recipe.

1 Preheat the oven to 400°F. Coat a roasting rack with cooking spray. Place the rack inside a large roasting pan.

2 Trim any excess fat from the tenderloin. Rub the tenderloin with the olive oil. Combine the breadcrumbs, parsley, garlic, pepper, and salt. Pat the breadcrumb mixture onto the tenderloin. Place the tenderloin on the prepared rack.

3 Roast the tenderloin for 20–25 minutes. Increase the temperature to 425°F and roast for 10–15 more minutes. Remove the roast from the oven, cover, and keep warm.

4 Whisk together the ingredients for the sauce in a small bowl.

5 Slice the tenderloin on the bias and serve with the sauce.

EXCHANGES/ CHOICES	Calories **155**	Sodium **195 mg**
	Calories from Fat **55**	Total Carbohydrate **7 g**
1/2 Carbohydrate	Total Fat **6.0 g**	Dietary Fiber **0 g**
3 Lean Meat	Saturated Fat **2.0 g**	Sugars **2 g**
	Trans Fat **0.0 g**	Protein **18 g**
	Cholesterol **50 mg**	

Roast Beef Hash

1/2 pound small red-skinned potatoes, cut into 1/4-inch pieces

2 carrots, peeled, quartered lengthwise, and thinly sliced

1 tablespoon, plus 2 teaspoons olive oil

1 medium onion, finely chopped

2 cloves garlic, minced

1 1/4 cups frozen corn

kosher salt, to taste

freshly ground black pepper, to taste

6 ounces cooked roast beef, cut into 1/3-inch pieces

For the ultimate comfort food, serve this slimmed down version of Roast Beef Hash to your friends and family. Frozen corn gives the hash color and provides extra fiber. I've always thought that hash was one of those sloppy messy foods that is perfect on the American table. To make this recipe super simple, purchase low-sodium roast beef at the deli counter.

1   Cook potatoes in a medium saucepan of boiling water for 4 minutes. Add carrots and cook 2 minutes longer. Drain.

2   Spray a large nonstick skillet with nonstick cooking spray. Add 1 tablespoon oil and heat over medium-low heat. Add onion and garlic to skillet and cook, stirring frequently, until onion is golden brown, about 7 minutes.

3   Increase heat to medium-high. Add remaining 2 teaspoons oil. Add potatoes, carrots, corn, salt, and pepper, and cook, stirring occasionally, until mixture starts to form a crust, about 10 minutes.

4   Stir in beef and press down on mixture to help form a crust. Cook until crusty on the bottom, about 5 minutes.

EXCHANGES/ CHOICES

1 1/2 Starch
1 Vegetable
2 Lean Meat
1 Fat

Calories **260**
    Calories from Fat **80**
Total Fat **9.0 g**
    Saturated Fat **2.0 g**
    Trans Fat **0.0 g**
Cholesterol **45 mg**

Sodium **45 mg**
Total Carbohydrate **28 g**
    Dietary Fiber **4 g**
    Sugars **5 g**
Protein **18 g**

Roast Beef Reubens

1/4 cup fat-free Thousand Island dressing

8 slices thin rye bread

1/2 pound sliced deli roast beef

1/2 cup jarred sauerkraut, drained

4 thin (3/4 ounce each) slices reduced-fat Swiss cheese

2 tsp margarine (60% vegetable oil), tub

Aaah, a Reuben. You'll be drawn into the richness of the dressing, the tang of the sauerkraut, the layers of roast beef, the melted cheese, and the crunch of the rye bread.

1 Spray a large nonstick skillet with butter-flavored nonstick spray, then heat over medium-low heat. Spread the dressing on the slices of bread. Top half of the slices with roast beef, sauerkraut, and a slice of cheese. Cover each slice with remaining bread.

2 Melt the butter in a large nonstick skillet over medium-low heat. When hot, add the sandwiches and toast on each side for 2 minutes. Cover and cook for 1–2 minutes until the cheese melts.

EXCHANGES/ CHOICES		
2 Starch	Calories **255**	Sodium **940 mg**
2 Lean Meat	Calories from Fat **55**	Total Carbohydrate **25 g**
1 Fat	Total Fat **8.0 g**	Dietary Fiber **6 g**
	Saturated Fat **3.0 g**	Sugars **4 g**
	Trans Fat **0.0 g**	Protein **21 g**
	Cholesterol **40 mg**	

Roast Chicken

1 (3–4 pound) roasting chicken

1/2 granny smith apple, unpeeled and chopped

1/2 yellow onion, peeled and coarsely chopped

1/2 head garlic, separated into cloves, skins left on

3 sprigs thyme, folded over

3 sprigs rosemary, folded over

kosher salt, to taste

freshly ground pepper, to taste

1 tablespoon olive oil

I've always taught that it's wise to learn solid basic culinary techniques rather than trying to learn a ton of recipes. Roast Chicken is one of those classic techniques that, once you know how to do it, will impress everyone you serve.

1 Preheat the oven to 475°F. Wash the chicken inside and out and pat dry.

2 In a bowl, combine the apple, onion, garlic, herbs, salt, pepper, and olive oil. Stuff the cavity of the chicken with this mixture. Tie the chicken using twine. First, tie the legs together and continue using the twine to bind the wings to the body of the chicken.

3 Rub the outside of the chicken on both sides with olive oil and sprinkle with salt and pepper. Place the chicken in a roasting pan sprayed with cooking spray, breast side down, uncovered, and roast for 45 minutes.

4 After 45 minutes, lower the temperature to 400°F, turn the chicken over on its back, and continue to roast for 30-40 minutes until the chicken juices run clear. The legs should move easily.

5 Remove the chicken from the oven and let rest on a platter, loosely covered for 20 minutes, to allow the juices to settle back into the chicken and to make carving easier. Remove the twine to carve. The stuffing does not get consumed, discard upon serving. (It is for flavoring purposes only.) Remove and discard skin. Store any leftovers in a covered container no more than 2 days.

EXCHANGES/ CHOICES		
2 Lean Meat	Calories **95**	Sodium **35 mg**
	Calories from Fat **40**	Total Carbohydrate **0 g**
	Total Fat **4.5 g**	Dietary Fiber **0 g**
	Saturated Fat **1.1 g**	Sugars **0 g**
	Trans Fat **0.0 g**	Protein **12 g**
	Cholesterol **35 mg**	

Spiced Beef Stew with Dried Fruits

1 tablespoon canola oil

2 pounds lean chuck roast, trimmed of fat, cut into 1-inch cubes

1 large onion, cut into thin slices

2 medium peeled carrots, sliced on a bias about 1/2-inch thick

2 tablespoons flour

1 teaspoon ground cumin

1/2 teaspoon ground coriander

1/4 teaspoon ground cinnamon

3/4 teaspoon salt

1/2 teaspoon black pepper

3 cups low-fat, reduced-sodium beef stock

1 28-ounce can crushed tomatoes

1/2 cup halved pitted dried apricots

1/2 cup halved pitted dried prunes

Beef stew was a staple in my home growing up. Unfortunately, as our family grew busier, we made a fatal error in judgment: we resorted to canned beef stew! How we ever thought this would be a substitute for my mom's wonderfully aromatic stew was beyond us. Fortunately, now I've brought it back and jazzed it up with some dried fruits. My Eastern European ancestors used to make it this way, so this recipe is in their honor.

1   Heat the oil in a large Dutch oven over medium-high heat. In several batches, add the beef and sauté for about 4–5 minutes until browned. Remove the beef from the pan.

2   In the drippings, sauté the onion and carrots for about 5 minutes. Add the beef back to the pan and sprinkle with flour, cumin, coriander, cinnamon, salt, and pepper and sauté for 1 minute.

3   Add in the beef stock and tomatoes and bring to a boil. Lower the heat, cover, and simmer for about 30–40 minutes. Add in the apricots and prunes and simmer another 30 minutes. Add in more stock if the mixture becomes too thick.

EXCHANGES/ CHOICES		
1 Fruit	Calories **240**	Sodium **560 mg**
2 Vegetable	Calories from Fat **65**	Total Carbohydrate **25 g**
3 Lean Meat	Total Fat **7.0 g**	Dietary Fiber **4 g**
	Saturated Fat **1.6 g**	Sugars **16 g**
	Trans Fat **0.0 g**	Protein **22 g**
	Cholesterol **55 mg**	

Slow Cooked BBQ Chicken

RUB

2 tablespoons paprika

1 tablespoon sugar

1 tablespoon chili powder (mild or hot)

2 teaspoons dried thyme

1 teaspoon onion powder

1 teaspoon dried oregano

1 teaspoon lemon pepper

1/4 teaspoon cayenne pepper

8 (3 1/2 ounces each) bone-in, skinless chicken thighs

1/3 cup unsweetened apple juice

BBQ SAUCE

1/2 cup low-sodium ketchup

1/3 cup red wine vinegar

1/2 medium (1 cup) onion, chopped

1 tablespoon brown sugar

2 teaspoons Worcestershire sauce

2 garlic cloves, minced

1/2 teaspoon liquid smoke flavoring

1/4 teaspoon fresh ground black pepper

The secret to moist delectable chicken on the grill is to slow cook it. So be patient, because it will be so worth it. The rub can be used for so many other grilled foods, so save some—it can be saved for up to a year. And be sure to add the BBQ sauce to the chicken at the very end of the cooking. Don't add it too early or you'll have burnt chicken!

1 Prepare the grill. For both gas and charcoal grills, coat the grill rack with cooking spray. Or, dip a large piece of paper towel into vegetable oil and hold it in a set of tongs. Rub the grill with the oil-soaked towel. For a gas grill, set one burner to medium, leave the remaining burners off. For a charcoal grill, arrange the coals so that one part of the fire is hotter than the other.

2 Combine all the rub ingredients. Rub the chicken and let the chicken stand at room temperature for 15 minutes so the rub has a chance to permeate the chicken.

3 Add the chicken to the grill rack set above the medium burners on a gas grill or on the cool side of charcoal grill away from the hot coals. Cover the grill. Maintain the grill temperature at about 300°F.

4 Baste each piece of chicken with some of the apple juice. Grill for about 45 minutes on one side, basting occasionally with apple juice. Turn the chicken thighs and continue to cook the chicken for about another 45 minutes, basting occasionally with the apple juice.

EXCHANGES/ CHOICES		
1 1/2 Carbohydrate	Calories **335**	Sodium **220 mg**
4 Lean Meat	Calories from Fat **115**	Total Carbohydrate **24 g**
1 Fat	Total Fat **13.0 g**	Dietary Fiber **3 g**
	Saturated Fat **3.5 g**	Sugars **17 g**
	Trans Fat **0.0 g**	Protein **31 g**
	Cholesterol **105 mg**	

5   While the chicken is grilling, combine all the ingredients for the BBQ sauce in a small saucepan. Bring to a boil, lower the heat, and simmer for 30 minutes.

6   Brush one side of the chicken with sauce and continue to cook, covered, for 5 minutes. Turn over each piece and brush with more sauce. Grill for another 5 minutes.

7   Remove all the chicken from the grill and serve with any additional heated sauce.

A Few Great Tips for Everyday American Cooking

Improve your cooking dramatically with some useful hints I've been teaching my cooking students for years. Your cooking doesn't need to get any more complex; learn to make simple foods better.

- Cook your onions more and your garlic less. Give onions time to develop their sweet flavor. Get the other vegetables going before you add garlic; it burns easily and can make your dish taste bitter if added too soon.

- Don't always go by the exact cook time a recipe calls for. Learn to recognize what "golden brown" or "reduced by half" looks like. Remember that your pan size and heat source may be different than the recipe you are following.

- Invest in a few really good pans. Spend what you can afford on heavy, flat-bottomed pots and pans that can go from stovetop to oven. Make sure there are lots of layers of construction in the pan so that it delivers even heat.

- Grind your own spices whenever you can. Buy cumin in seed form and grind in a coffee.grinder right before adding to your recipe. It makes a major difference in flavor.

- Use vegetable or chicken stock instead of water to boil grains and cook pasta. It adds a wonderful richness to the simplest of foods.

- Add a splash of vinegar or citrus juice to almost any vegetable dish at the end of the cooking to brighten it and intensify the flavor.

- Although you might want to skip the parsley garnish, don't. The humblest of food can be elevated to new heights with the simple addition of chopped parsley.

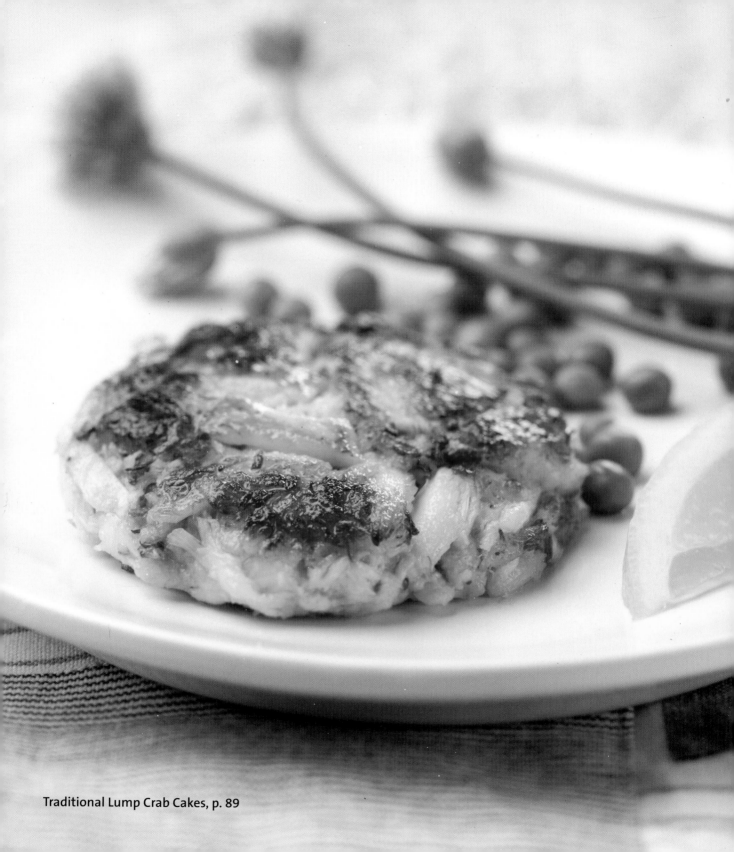

Traditional Lump Crab Cakes, p. 89

Traditional Lump Crab Cakes

1 pound lump crabmeat, picked over to remove any cartilage and shells

3 tablespoons light mayonnaise (such as Hellmann's Light)

3 tablespoons dry breadcrumbs

2 tablespoons Dijon mustard

3 tablespoons minced scallions

1 tablespoon minced parsley

1 teaspoon Old Bay seasoning

1/4 teaspoon crushed red pepper flakes

1 egg

3 tablespoons all-purpose flour

1 tablespoon canola oil

For delicious, fresh crab cakes, look no further than your own kitchen. Be sure to splurge on jumbo lump crabmeat. This crab cake is all about the crab and has just enough breading and mayo to bind it together. Refrigerating for a half hour is really what keeps these minimally breaded crab cakes together and makes them supremely delicious.

1   Combine all ingredients except the flour and canola oil in a large bowl and mix well. Shape the mixture into 7 crab cakes and set on a plate. Cover and refrigerate for 30 minutes to set.

2   Heat the canola oil in a large 12-inch skillet (preferably cast iron) over medium heat. Dredge each crab cake with flour to lightly coat both sides. Add the cakes to the skillet and cook for about 4–5 minutes per side. Drain on paper towels.

EXCHANGES/ CHOICES		
1/2 Carbohydrate	Calories **135**	Sodium **470 mg**
2 Lean Meat	Calories from Fat **55**	Total Carbohydrate **6 g**
1/2 Fat	Total Fat **6.0 g**	Dietary Fiber **0 g**
	Saturated Fat **0.9 g**	Sugars **1 g**
	Trans Fat **0.0 g**	Protein **14 g**
	Cholesterol **120 mg**	

Turkey Pesto Sandwiches

1/4 cup fat-free mayonnaise

1 1/2 tablespoon prepared pesto

1 teaspoon lemon juice

1/2 teaspoon dried oregano

1/8 teaspoon fresh ground black pepper

4 6-inch French rolls (preferably whole-wheat), cut in half lengthwise

1/2 pound sliced cooked lean turkey breast

8 slices tomato

8 fresh arugula or spinach leaves

1 1/2 ounces thinly sliced part-skim mozzarella cheese

I have clients who, if I let them, would eat a turkey sandwich every day. What a rut! So I developed something a bit jazzier than two slices of bread with turkey in between. Just a small tad of pesto livens up an everyday lunch with great taste in each bite.

1 Preheat the oven to 350°F. Mix the mayonnaise, pesto, lemon juice, dried oregano, and pepper in a small bowl.

2 Put the cut rolls on a baking sheet. Place in the oven for 5 minutes, then remove.

3 Preheat the broiler. Spread the pesto mixture evenly between the French rolls.

4 Layer the turkey, tomato, arugula or spinach, and mozzarella cheese on the rolls.

5 Place the sandwiches on a baking sheet and broil for 2 minutes until cheese is melted.

EXCHANGES/ CHOICES		
3 Starch 3 Lean Meat	Calories **375** Calories from Fat **80** Total Fat **9.0 g** Saturated Fat **2.4 g** Trans Fat **0.0 g** Cholesterol **35 mg**	Sodium **1145 mg** Total Carbohydrate **52 g** Dietary Fiber **8 g** Sugars **10 g** Protein **25 g**

SERVES 6 SERVING SIZE 2/3 cup PREPARATION TIME 15 minutes COOK TIME 15 minutes

Turkey Stroganoff

8 ounces egg noodles

2 teaspoons poppy seeds

12 ounces fresh roasted turkey breast, cut into 2 × 1/2-inch strips

salt, to taste

1/2 teaspoon freshly ground black pepper

2 (4 ounces each) Portobello mushrooms

1 small red onion, thinly sliced

1 tablespoon butter

1 1/2 tablespoons all-purpose flour

1 1/2 cups reduced-sodium beef broth

1/2 cup reduced-fat sour cream

1 1/2 teaspoons Dijon mustard

In the 1960s we cooked noodles, added cooked ground beef, made a creamy sauce, and mixed them together and that was the standard dinner of the times. But I like to think that a good stroganoff hasn't completely disappeared from the dinner table. My secret to a hearty stroganoff: Use fresh roasted turkey breast in place of beef and Portobello mushrooms in place of regular button mushrooms and watch requests for this dish go up tenfold.

1 Cook noodles according to package directions. Toss noodles with poppy seeds and return to empty cooking pot to keep warm. Sprinkle turkey strips with salt and pepper; toss to coat. Remove and discard stems from mushrooms. Cut mushroom caps into quarters and thinly slice.

2 Meanwhile, lightly coat large nonstick skillet with nonstick cooking spray and set over medium-high heat. Sauté onion 2 minutes. Add mushrooms and sauté until mushrooms are tender, about 5–6 minutes. Transfer to large bowl.

3 Melt butter in skillet over medium heat. Add flour and cook for 1 minute, continuously stirring. Gradually whisk in broth. Cook, stirring with wooden spoon, until sauce thickens and boils, about 4 minutes.

4 Reduce heat to low. Blend in sour cream and mustard. Return turkey and reserved vegetables with accumulated juices to skillet. Cook until heated through (do not boil). Divide noodles among plates and spoon stroganoff on top.

EXCHANGES/CHOICES

2 Starch
3 Lean Meat

Calories **285**
  Calories from Fat **65**
Total Fat **7.0 g**
  Saturated Fat **3.2 g**
  Trans Fat **0.0 g**
Cholesterol **90 mg**

Sodium **205 mg**
Total Carbohydrate **31 g**
  Dietary Fiber **2 g**
  Sugars **3 g**
Protein **25 g**

Vegetable Provençal Tart, p. 109

CHAPTER 5
International

Chicken Cacciatore | 94

Chicken Paprikash | 95

Chinese Five-Spice Steak with Chinese Noodles | 96

Falafel | 97

Gnocchi with Tomatoes, Chickpeas, and Spinach | 98

Greek Lamb Chops | 99

Grilled Pork and Cheese Quesadillas | 101

Indian Lamb Curry | 102

Jamaican Chicken Thighs | 103

Malaysian Shrimp with Pineapple | 104

Provençal Fish Stew | 106

Spanish Chicken with Red Peppers | 107

Sweet and Sour Pork | 108

Vegetable Provençal Tart | 109

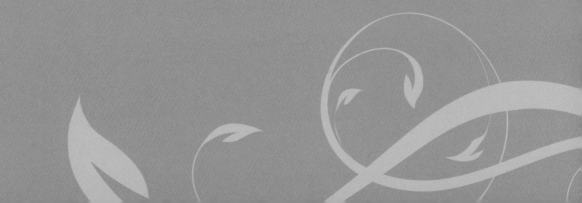

Chicken Cacciatore

8 (4 ounces each) skin on, bone-in chicken thighs

kosher salt, to taste

freshly ground black pepper, to taste

1 teaspoon olive oil

1 large onion, chopped

8 ounces button mushrooms, sliced

3 garlic cloves, minced

2 tablespoons all-purpose flour

1 cup dry red wine (dry Chianti works well)

1/2 cup low-fat, reduced-sodium chicken broth

2 14 1/2-ounce cans diced tomatoes, undrained

1 tablespoon fresh minced thyme

1 cup fresh chopped basil

Some American versions of this traditional Italian comfort dish don't quite get it right. True chicken cacciatore is a smooth tomato wine sauce flavored with only onion, mushrooms, and garlic. To keep the chicken moist, sauté it with the skin on, but remove it for the final simmer. Keep the flavor in without unnecessary fat. This recipe works best with chicken thighs.

1 Season the chicken with salt and pepper. Heat the oil in a large sauté pan or Dutch oven on medium-high heat until shimmering and almost smoking. Add the chicken in two batches, skin side down, until well browned, about 5–6 minutes. Turn over the thighs and brown for another 5–6 minutes. Repeat with the second batch of chicken. Remove the chicken to a plate.

2 Drain off all but 2 teaspoons of the fat. Add the onion and mushrooms to the pan and sauté minimally for about 10 minutes. Add the garlic and sauté until fragrant, about 30 seconds. Sprinkle the onion and mushrooms with the flour until the flour is incorporated into the vegetables, about 30 seconds.

3 Add in the wine, broth, and tomatoes and bring to a boil. Remove the skin from each piece of chicken. Discard the skin. Add the chicken to the pan, nestling it in the sauce. Lower the heat and simmer the chicken for about 30 minutes. Remove the chicken from the sauce, place on a plate, and tent with foil. Raise the heat and add the thyme and additional salt and pepper, as desired. Cook for 3–4 minutes until thick. Add in the fresh basil. Serve the sauce over the chicken.

EXCHANGES/ CHOICES		
4 Vegetable	Calories **330**	Sodium **450 mg**
3 Lean Meat	Calories from Fat **115**	Total Carbohydrate **20 g**
2 Fat	Total Fat **13.0 g**	Dietary Fiber **4 g**
	Saturated Fat **3.5 g**	Sugars **9 g**
	Trans Fat **0.0 g**	Protein **30 g**
	Cholesterol **90 mg**	

Chicken Paprikash

8 ounces uncooked egg
  noodles

2 teaspoons vegetable oil

1 medium onion, halved
  and thinly sliced

1 pound boneless, skinless
  chicken breasts

2 tablespoons sweet
  Hungarian paprika,
  divided

1/2 cup low-fat, reduced-
  sodium chicken broth

1/2 cup low-fat sour cream

1/2 cup nonfat sour cream

1/4 teaspoon kosher salt

1/4 teaspoon freshly
  ground black pepper

I'm half Hungarian, so one would hope a good paprikash recipe was handed down to me. And indeed one was. But with a few tweaks here and there, I transformed it into a much healthier dish than my ancestors' original recipe.

1 Cook egg noodles according to package directions. Meanwhile, heat the oil in a large skillet over medium heat. Add the onion and sauté for 3–5 minutes, or until the onion softens and turns golden.

2 Coat both sides of the chicken with 1 tablespoon of the paprika. Add the chicken to the skillet and sauté on both sides for a total of 10 minutes.

3 Add the chicken broth, using a wooden spoon to scrape the bottom of the pan. Bring to a simmer, and cook over medium heat to reduce the broth, about 3 minutes. Stir the paprika into the sour creams. Add the salt and pepper. Add the sour cream mixture to the chicken and heat through, without allowing the mixture to boil. Serve over cooked egg noodles.

EXCHANGES/ CHOICES		
2 1/2 Starch	Calories **445**	Sodium **310 mg**
1/2 Carbohydrate	Calories from Fat **100**	Total Carbohydrate **50 g**
4 Lean Meat	Total Fat **11.0 g**	Dietary Fiber **4 g**
1/2 Fat	Saturated Fat **3.8 g**	Sugars **6 g**
	Trans Fat **0.1 g**	Protein **35 g**
	Cholesterol **125 mg**	

Chinese Five-Spice Steak with Chinese Noodles

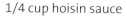

1/4 cup hoisin sauce

1 tablespoon reduced-sodium soy sauce

1 teaspoon Chinese five-spice powder

1 pound flank steak, trimmed and cut on the bias into thin slices

2 teaspoons peanut oil

2 tablespoons minced scallions

3 garlic cloves, minced

1 tomato, cut into 6 wedges

1 tablespoon fresh basil, minced

8 ounces cooked Chinese noodles

I got hooked on Chinese five-spice while traveling in China several years ago. I was told this blend of exotic spices, including cinnamon and Szechuan peppercorns, is used every day to bring complex flavors to the simplest of foods. This homey stir-fry is simple to prepare, but tastes like you've been cooking all day.

1   Combine the hoisin sauce, soy sauce, and Chinese five-spice in a zippered plastic bag. Add the flank steak and turn to coat. Marinate the steak in the refrigerator for 2–24 hours.

2   After the steak has marinated, remove from the refrigerator and let the steak come to room temperature. Drain the marinade from the steak.

3   Heat the oil in a wok or heavy skillet over medium-high heat. Add the scallions and garlic and stir-fry for 30 seconds. Add the beef and stir-fry for 5–6 minutes. Add the tomato and basil and stir-fry for 2 minutes. Serve over Chinese noodles.

EXCHANGES/ CHOICES

1 1/2 Starch
3 Lean Meat
1/2 Fat

Calories **275**
    Calories from Fat **90**
Total Fat **10.0 g**
    Saturated Fat **3.1 g**
    Trans Fat **0.0 g**
Cholesterol **55 mg**

Sodium **285 mg**
Total Carbohydrate **20 g**
    Dietary Fiber **1 g**
    Sugars **4 g**
Protein **26 g**

Falafel

1 15-ounce can chickpeas, drained and rinsed

1 teaspoon olive oil

1/2 teaspoon ground cumin

pinch of cayenne pepper

pinch of turmeric

1 garlic clove, crushed

1 tablespoon lemon juice

1 medium carrot, finely grated

1 tablespoon chopped fresh cilantro

SAUCE

1/2 cup plain nonfat Greek yogurt

2 teaspoons sesame tahini

1 teaspoon fresh lemon juice

2 tablespoons chopped fresh mint

1 teaspoon water

dash cayenne

sea salt, to taste

freshly ground black pepper, to taste

4 medium whole-wheat pita breads

1 heart of romaine lettuce, shredded

2 plum tomatoes, thinly sliced

Long before I ever traveled to the Middle East, my mom prepared homemade falafel for our family. While other families served soups and stews for comfort food, the first choice to soothe us was Mom's falafel. Thanks Mom!

1 Preheat the oven to 400°F. Line a baking sheet with baking parchment. Put the chickpeas in a bowl with the oil and use a potato masher to mash them until smooth. Mix in the cumin, cayenne pepper, turmeric, garlic, lemon juice, carrot, cilantro, and salt and pepper to taste. Alternatively, mix all the ingredients, except the carrot and cilantro, in a food processor. Transfer the mixture to a bowl and stir in the carrot and cilantro.

2 Shape the mixture into 16 flat, round patties, each about 1 1/4 inches across, and place them on the parchment-lined baking sheet. Bake for 15–20 minutes or until crisp and lightly browned, turning them over halfway through the cooking time.

3 About 3 minutes before the falafels have finished cooking, put the pita breads in the oven to warm. Split the breads in half widthwise and gently open out each half to make a pocket.

4 Half-fill the pita bread pockets with the shredded lettuce and sliced tomatoes, then divide the falafels among them. Mix together the yogurt, tahini, lemon juice, mint, cayenne, salt, and pepper to taste, and drizzle over the falafels. Serve hot.

EXCHANGES/ CHOICES			
3 Starch	Calories **325**		Sodium **440 mg**
1 Vegetable	Calories from Fat **55**		Total Carbohydrate **56 g**
1 Lean Meat	Total Fat **6.0 g**		Dietary Fiber **12 g**
1/2 Fat	Saturated Fat **0.8 g**		Sugars **8 g**
	Trans Fat **0.0 g**		Protein **16 g**
	Cholesterol **0 mg**		

Gnocchi with Tomatoes, Chickpeas, and Spinach

1 pound commercially prepared whole-wheat gnocchi

1 tablespoon olive oil

1 15-ounce can chickpeas, drained and rinsed

1 14 1/2-ounce can diced tomatoes

6 cups fresh baby spinach leaves

This gnocchi cooks up pillowy soft and the slightly sticky texture holds on to the simple tomato sauce. Perfectly prepared gnocchi are the ultimate comfort food from Italy.

1   Bring a large saucepan of lightly salted water to a boil. Add the gnocchi and cook until they float, about 3–5 minutes. Drain and set aside.

2   Meanwhile, heat the oil in a large skillet over medium heat. Add the chickpeas and canned tomatoes and cook for 3–4 minutes. Add the cooked gnocchi and toss gently to coat.

3   Add the spinach and cook, gently stirring, for about 2 minutes until spinach is wilted. Serve immediately.

*Recipe courtesy of Janel Ovrut, MS, RD

EXCHANGES/CHOICES		
2 1/2 Starch 1 Vegetable	Calories **225** Calories from Fat **30** Total Fat **3.5 g** Saturated Fat **0.5 g** Trans Fat **0.0 g** Cholesterol **0 mg**	Sodium **420 mg** Total Carbohydrate **44 g** Dietary Fiber **9 g** Sugars **4 g** Protein **6 g**

Garlic has got to be the most prevalent staple in kitchens around the world. Here are some garlic tips to help you know how to select, handle, and store it to get the best flavor.

- Buy firm, plump heavy heads with tight papery skins. The heavier the garlic is, the juicier and better tasting it will be.

- Avoid garlic with mold, green sprouts, or sunken cloves. All are signs of deterioration.

- Store garlic in a cool, dry place, not in the refrigerator. Discard when it begins to feel soft.

- Set the garlic head on a flat surface and use the heel of your hand to press down until the cloves separate.

- To peel garlic, break the skin with the flat side of a knife. Use just enough pressure to crack the skin, not smash the clove.

- If you have to peel a lot of garlic, drop a whole bunch of heads into boiling water and blanch for 10 seconds. Drain and peel.

Greek Lamb Chops

3 teaspoons fresh lemon juice

2 teaspoons dried oregano leaves

2 teaspoons minced garlic

1/2 teaspoon kosher salt

1/4 teaspoon freshly ground black pepper

4 (3 ounces each) lean boneless loin lamb chops, trimmed of fat

The first memory I have of really good lamb chops was on my first visit to Greece many years ago. Fresh lemon juice, garlic, and oregano add tons of flavor to the lamb. While you might not be able to hop a plane to Greece tomorrow, bring a little bit of it into your home with this wonderful dish.

1 In a small bowl, combine the lemon juice, oregano, garlic, salt, and pepper. Mix well.

2 Place the lamb chops on a broiler pan. Rub each side of the lamb chops with the garlic oregano mixture. Broil about 4 inches from the heat for about 4–5 minutes per side until cooked to your liking.

EXCHANGES/CHOICES

3 Lean Meat

Calories **125**
Calories from Fat **45**
Total Fat **5.0 g**
Saturated Fat **2.0 g**
Trans Fat **0.0 g**
Cholesterol **55 mg**

Sodium **285 mg**
Total Carbohydrate **1 g**
Dietary Fiber **0 g**
Sugars **0 g**
Protein **18 g**

Oregano is indispensable in many cuisines across the world. It is used throughout the Middle East, Mexico, and Mediterranean countries. With such a robust flavor, peppery bite, and zing, it really makes dishes sparkle. Here's how to get the most out of oregano in your cooking.

• Oregano is excellent when it is dried.

• You will most likely find dried Greek oregano and dried Mexican oregano. Use Greek oregano in Mediterranean dishes where the flavors are more subtle, and Mexican oregano in spicier foods, as its flavor is more pronounced and intense.

• If you have an excess of fresh oregano from your summer garden, you can dry the leaves. Just tie the stems together and hang in a warm, dry well ventilated place.

• Add dried oregano to the woody flavor of sautéed mushrooms.

• Add a few fresh oregano leaves to a tossed salad.

Grilled Pork and Cheese Quesadillas, p. 101

Grilled Pork and Cheese Quesadillas

1 teaspoon olive oil

1/2 cup minced onion

2 teaspoons minced garlic

1 pound ground pork loin

8 6-inch corn or whole-
wheat tortillas

1 cup reduced-fat Mexican
cheese blend

3 scallions, thinly sliced

1 3-ounce can chopped
mild or hot green chilies

GARNISH

1/2 cup nonfat Greek
yogurt

1/2 cup prepared mild or
hot salsa

1 cup diced tomatoes

A Mexican favorite can now be yours. When a quesadilla is grilled rather than prepared in an indoor oven, the result is smoky, rich-flavored quesadilla. If you can't grill outside, this works great prepared on a stovetop grill pan.

1   Prepare an outdoor grill for medium heat. Heat the oil in a large skillet over medium heat. Add the onion and sauté for 3 minutes. Add the garlic and sauté for 1 minute. Add the pork and sauté for 5–6 minutes. Drain any excess fat.

2   On two baking sheets, lay out 4 tortillas. Spray tops lightly with oil. Flip over. Spread 1/2 cup of pork evenly over the tortilla. Sprinkle with cheese, scallions, and chilies. Top all the tortillas with the remaining tortillas to form a quesadilla and press together lightly. Spray lightly with oil.

3   When the grill is hot, place quesadillas on the grill. Grill for 5–7 minutes on each side. During some of this time, you may cover the grill to help melt the cheese and brown the quesadillas. When the first side is golden, flip over and grill the other side. Cut into wedges and serve with yogurt, salsa, and tomatoes.

EXCHANGES/ CHOICES		
1/2 Starch	Calories **185**	Sodium **265 mg**
1 Vegetable	Calories from Fat **55**	Total Carbohydrate **16 g**
2 Lean Meat	Total Fat **6.0 g**	Dietary Fiber **3 g**
1/2 Fat	Saturated Fat **2.2 g**	Sugars **3 g**
	Trans Fat **0.0 g**	Protein **18 g**
	Cholesterol **40 mg**	

Indian Lamb Curry

1 teaspoon olive oil

12 ounces well-trimmed boneless lamb loin, cut into 3/4-inch chunks

1 medium onion, finely chopped

4 cloves garlic, minced

1 tablespoon grated fresh ginger

1 tablespoon curry powder

4 cups cauliflower florets

1 cup no-salt-added canned crushed tomatoes

salt, to taste

2 cups water

1/4 cup golden raisins

1 1/2 cups frozen peas

1/3 cup chopped cilantro

2 tablespoons flour

2 tablespoons water

1/2 cup plain nonfat Greek yogurt

Perfectly cooked cauliflower and tender chunks of lamb in a thick and luscious curry sauce will satisfy your cravings for a different weeknight meal.

1 Heat oil in Dutch oven over medium heat. Add lamb and cook until browned, about 5 minutes. With slotted spoon, transfer lamb to bowl or plate.

2 Add onion, garlic, and ginger to pan and cook, stirring frequently, until onion is tender, about 5 minutes. Add curry powder and cauliflower, stirring to coat.

3 Add tomatoes, salt, and water to pan and bring to a boil. Return lamb to pan and reduce to a simmer. Cover and cook until lamb and cauliflower are tender, about 40 minutes.

4 Add the raisins, peas, and cilantro, and cook until peas are heated through, about 3 minutes. Stir flour and water together in small bowl. Add to the lamb and simmer for 5 minutes, until slightly thickened. Turn off the heat and stir the yogurt into pan.

EXCHANGES/ CHOICES		
1 Carbohydrate 2 Lean Meat	Calories **155** Calories from Fat **40**	Sodium **70 mg** Total Carbohydrate **16 g**
	Total Fat **4.5 g** Saturated Fat **1.6 g** Trans Fat **0.0 g**	Dietary Fiber **4 g** Sugars **7 g**
	Cholesterol **35 mg**	Protein **13 g**

Jamaican Chicken Thighs

RUB

1 tablespoon garlic powder

2 teaspoons onion powder

2 teaspoons allspice

1 teaspoon thyme leaves

1 teaspoon ground ginger

1/2 teaspoon ground
nutmeg

1/2 teaspoon cayenne
pepper

1/4 teaspoon salt

1/8 teaspoon freshly
ground black pepper

6 skinless, bone-in chicken
thighs

2 teaspoons canola oil

This flavorful dish will transport you to a more exotic location, without ever leaving your kitchen. Make this rub as spicy as you desire. The rub is great for so many other foods, such as flank steak or pork tenderloin. Make the rub and store it for no more than 1 year.

1 Preheat the oven to 350°F. Line a baking sheet with foil or parchment paper. Set aside.

2 Combine the rub ingredients in a small bowl. Coat both sides of the chicken thighs with the rub.

3 Heat the canola oil in a 12-inch skillet over medium-high heat. Add the chicken thighs and cook one side for 5 minutes. Turn and continue to cook on the other side for about 3–4 minutes.

4 Remove the chicken from the skillet and place on the prepared baking sheet. Continue to roast the chicken in the oven for 20 minutes or until chicken is cooked through and no traces of pink remain. The juices should run clear.

EXCHANGES/ CHOICES		
2 Lean Meat 1/2 Fat	Calories **125**	Sodium **140 mg**
	Calories from Fat **65**	Total Carbohydrate **3 g**
	Total Fat **7.0 g**	Dietary Fiber **0 g**
	Saturated Fat **1.7 g**	Sugars **1 g**
	Trans Fat **0.0 g**	Protein **13 g**
	Cholesterol **45 mg**	

Malaysian Shrimp with Pineapple

2 teaspoons canola oil

1 onion, thinly sliced

3 garlic cloves, minced

1 teaspoon ground cumin

1 teaspoon turmeric

1 teaspoon ground coriander

1/8 to 1/4 teaspoon crushed red pepper flakes

2 tablespoons light soy sauce

1 tablespoon light brown sugar

1/3 cup light coconut milk

1 pound large shrimp, peeled and deveined

2 cups fresh pineapple chunks

2 scallions, thinly sliced

Take a spin on the exotic side with this coriander and cumin scented shrimp dish. The shrimp are bathed in a slightly sweet sauce with the delightful creaminess from the coconut milk. Try this dish with sea scallops, too.

1 Heat the oil in a wok or heavy skillet over medium-high heat. Add the onion and garlic and stir-fry for 5 minutes until the onion begins to soften. Add the cumin, turmeric, coriander, and red pepper flakes. Stir-fry for 2 minutes.

2 Whisk together the soy sauce, brown sugar, and coconut milk in a small bowl and add to the wok. Lower the heat, cover, and simmer for 5 minutes.

3 Add the shrimp into the sauce and simmer gently, uncovered, for 3–4 minutes until the shrimp are almost cooked through.

4 Add in the pineapple and scallions and cook for 1 minute.

EXCHANGES/ CHOICES		

1 Fruit
1 Vegetable
2 Lean Meat
	Calories **180**
	  Calories from Fat **40**
	Total Fat **4.5 g**
	  Saturated Fat **1.1 g**
	  Trans Fat **0.0 g**
	Cholesterol **130 mg**
		Sodium **450 mg**
		Total Carbohydrate **20 g**
		  Dietary Fiber **2 g**
		  Sugars **14 g**
		Protein **16 g**

Asian Flavors

Asian-flavored recipes call for a pantry stocked with a few bold ingredients. Here are some staples to have on hand to bring out the best of Asian-inspired recipes in your kitchen:

GINGER

Fresh ginger is a cornerstone of true Asian cooking. Good ginger is rock hard, with a skin that is taut across the bulb and looks shiny. You don't need to peel ginger if you are using it in a marinade.

The best way to grate ginger is to purchase a micro plane or ginger grater. A micro plane allows you to grate the ginger into a paste but does not capture the ginger juices. A traditional ginger grater is usually made of porcelain. You can grate ginger on its grating holes. The holes are surrounded by a well that captures the ginger juices, which can then be added back to your recipe for delicious flavor.

SCALLIONS

Scallions are very important to Asian cooking. For best results, smash the scallion pieces with the broad side of a knife to release its flavor before you chop it. Use the whole length of a scallion except for its bearded root and any straggly stalks.

SOY SAUCE

Soy sauce is the most critical ingredient in Asian cooking. Buy low-sodium varieties that are brewed. Non-brewed soy sauces contain way too many chemicals. Buy and taste several before you decide what you like.

SIMPLE ASIAN ADD-INS

- Add grated ginger and scallions to homemade or canned chicken broth to enhance flavor.

- Julienne ginger and scallions to top fish filets before cooking.

- Add soy sauce, minced ginger, and scallions to your favorite meatloaf recipe.

- Stuff a chicken with slices of ginger before roasting.

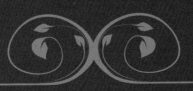

Provençal Fish Stew

2 teaspoons olive oil

1 large onion, chopped

3 garlic cloves, minced

2 celery stalks, minced

1 28-ounce can whole tomatoes, undrained

1 cup low-fat, reduced-sodium chicken broth

1/2 cup dry white wine

2 tablespoons tomato paste

1 teaspoon sweet paprika

1 teaspoon dried thyme

1/2 teaspoon celery seed

1 bay leaf

1/4 teaspoon cayenne pepper

1 pound cod, skinned, and cubed into 1 1/2-inch pieces

3/4 pound large shrimp, peeled and deveined, tails left on or off

1/2 cup fresh chopped basil

sea salt, to taste

freshly ground black pepper, to taste

France's fish stews are the ultimate comfort food. A hearty bowl of stew just needs a chunk of whole-grain bread and you have a meal.

1 Heat the oil in a large saucepan over medium-high heat. Add the onion, garlic, and celery and sauté for 5 minutes.

2 Add the whole tomatoes and juices to a large bowl. Crush the tomatoes with your hands until coarsely chopped. Add the tomatoes, broth, wine, tomato paste, paprika, dried thyme, celery seed, bay leaf, and cayenne pepper to the pot. Bring to a boil, lower the heat, and simmer uncovered for about 30–35 minutes.

3 Add the cod and shrimp to the pot and raise the heat to medium. Cook 5 minutes or until the cod is opaque and the shrimp turn pink. Turn off heat, discard the bay leaf, and add in the basil, salt, and pepper.

EXCHANGES/ CHOICES		
2 Vegetable 2 Lean Meat	Calories **145** Calories from Fat **20** Total Fat **2.5 g** Saturated Fat **0.4 g** Trans Fat **0.0 g** Cholesterol **85 mg**	Sodium **390 mg** Total Carbohydrate **10 g** Dietary Fiber **2 g** Sugars **5 g** Protein **20 g**

Spanish Chicken with Red Peppers

1 pound boneless, skinless chicken thighs

kosher salt, to taste

freshly ground black pepper, to taste

3 teaspoons olive oil, divided

2 large onions, halved and thinly sliced

2 medium red bell peppers, thinly sliced

1/4 cup diced prosciutto

2 garlic cloves, minced

1/2 teaspoon smoked paprika

1 14 1/2-ounce can diced tomatoes, undrained

10 pitted black olives, halved

1/4 cup finely minced parsley

Smoked paprika is the ultimate comfort food spice in Spain. It's easy to find in the grocery or specialty food markets, as well as by mail order. The smoky aroma of chicken and vegetables all simmering together is one-pot comfort.

1 Sprinkle the chicken thighs with salt and pepper. Heat 2 teaspoons of the olive oil in a large skillet over medium-high heat. Add the chicken thighs and sear on both sides for about 5 minutes per side. Remove the chicken from the skillet and set aside.

2 Add the remaining 1 teaspoon of olive oil to the skillet. Add in the onions, peppers, and prosciutto and sauté for about 10 minutes. Add in the garlic and paprika and sauté for 2 minutes. Add in the tomatoes and bring to a boil.

3 Add back the chicken, cover, and reduce heat to low. Simmer for about 10 minutes. Uncover and cook over high heat until most of the liquid evaporates. Add in the olives and parsley and heat through.

EXCHANGES/ CHOICES		
3 Vegetable	Calories **295**	Sodium **380 mg**
3 Lean Meat	Calories from Fat **125**	Total Carbohydrate **21 g**
2 Fat	Total Fat **14.0 g**	Dietary Fiber **5 g**
	Saturated Fat **3.2 g**	Sugars **10 g**
	Trans Fat **0.0 g**	Protein **24 g**
	Cholesterol **75 mg**	

Sweet and Sour Pork

SAUCE

1/2 cup unsweetened
  pineapple juice

5 tablespoons red wine
  vinegar

2 tablespoons sugar

2 teaspoons reduced-
  sodium soy sauce

2 teaspoons fresh peeled
  grated ginger

2 garlic cloves, minced

2 tablespoons tomato
  sauce

1/2 teaspoon
  Worcestershire sauce

1 tablespoon cornstarch or
  arrowroot

2 teaspoons canola or
  peanut oil, divided

3/4 pound lean pork
  tenderloin, cut into
  3/4-inch cubes

1/2 large red onion, thinly
  sliced

1 red bell pepper, cored,
  seeded, and thinly sliced

1 green bell pepper, cored,
  seeded, and thinly sliced

1/2 cup canned (water-
  packed) or fresh
  pineapple chunks

When I was in Asia, I discovered just how light and tasty sweet and sour dishes could be. Honestly, I always avoided ordering them in America; the overwhelming sweet taste and high-fat content just doesn't work for me. After that trip I developed a recipe reminiscent of what I tasted overseas: delightfully healthy with a balanced sweet and sour flavor.

1 To prepare the sauce, combine all the sauce ingredients in a measuring cup or small bowl and whisk together until combined. Set aside.

2 Heat 1 teaspoon of the oil in a large wok over medium-high heat. Add the pork and stir-fry for about 4–5 minutes, until pork is cooked through. Remove the pork from the wok. Add the remaining 1 teaspoon of oil and add in the onion and pepper. Stir-fry for about 5 minutes until the vegetables soften.

3 Add back the pork and the sauce. Mix well. Cook for 1 minute until sauce thickens. Add in the pineapple chunks.

EXCHANGES/ CHOICES		
1 1/2 Carbohydrate	Calories **205**	Sodium **180 mg**
2 Lean Meat	Calories from Fat **40**	Total Carbohydrate **23 g**
	Total Fat **4.5 g**	Dietary Fiber **2 g**
	Saturated Fat **1.0 g**	Sugars **15 g**
	Trans Fat **0.0 g**	Protein **18 g**
	Cholesterol **45 mg**	

Vegetable Provençal Tart

nonstick cooking spray

1 large sweet Vidalia onion, halved and sliced into 1/3-inch pieces

1 teaspoon good-quality balsamic vinegar

1 1/2 cups all-purpose flour

1 1/2 teaspoons chopped fresh thyme

1/2 teaspoon kosher salt, divided

1/3 cup ice water

2 tablespoons olive oil

1 tablespoon Dijon mustard

1 medium (8 ounces) zucchini, cut diagonally into 1/8-inch long slices

1/2 teaspoon black pepper, divided

2 medium tomatoes, cut into 1/4-inch slices

2 tablespoons freshly grated Parmesan cheese

1/4 cup chopped fresh basil

A friend of mine owns a cooking school in Arles, France, and each time I visit, she makes me her fabulous vegetable tart. Hers is a bit higher in fat, but I trimmed it down a bit. All the flavor, but not all the fat.

1   Coat large nonstick skillet with nonstick cooking spray and set over medium-high heat until hot. Reduce heat to medium-low and sauté onion until very soft and golden, about 20 minutes. Add the balsamic vinegar and sauté for another 5 minutes. Transfer to plate.

2   Preheat oven to 400°F. Mix flour, thyme, and 1/4 teaspoon salt in a large bowl. Stir in water and oil, just until a soft dough forms. Lightly sprinkle work surface with flour and roll out dough with a rolling pin into a 16 × 10-inch rectangle or 13-inch round. Fold in half and transfer to 12 × 6-inch tart pan or 9-inch round tart pan with removable bottom. Trim the edges. Spread the Dijon mustard evenly over the bottom of the tart with the back of a spoon.

3   Lightly coat skillet again with nonstick cooking spray and set over medium heat. Add zucchini to the skillet with 1/4 teaspoon black pepper and sauté until golden, 5–7 minutes.

4   Arrange a layer of tomatoes, followed by the zucchini, another layer of the remaining tomatoes, and the onion, overlapping them slightly on the bottom of the tart. Sprinkle with remaining 1/4 teaspoon salt, 1/4 teaspoon black pepper, and the Parmesan cheese. Bake for about 20 minutes until tart is a lightly golden brown. Remove from the oven and sprinkle the top with the basil and return to the oven for 3 more minutes. Let the tart cool for 5 minutes, then slice into wedges and serve.

EXCHANGES/ CHOICES		
1 Starch	Calories **150**	Sodium **185 mg**
1 Vegetable	Calories from Fat **40**	Total Carbohydrate **25 g**
1 Fat	Total Fat **4.5 g**	Dietary Fiber **2 g**
	Saturated Fat **0.8 g**	Sugars **5 g**
	Trans Fat **0.0 g**	Protein **4 g**
	Cholesterol **0 mg**	

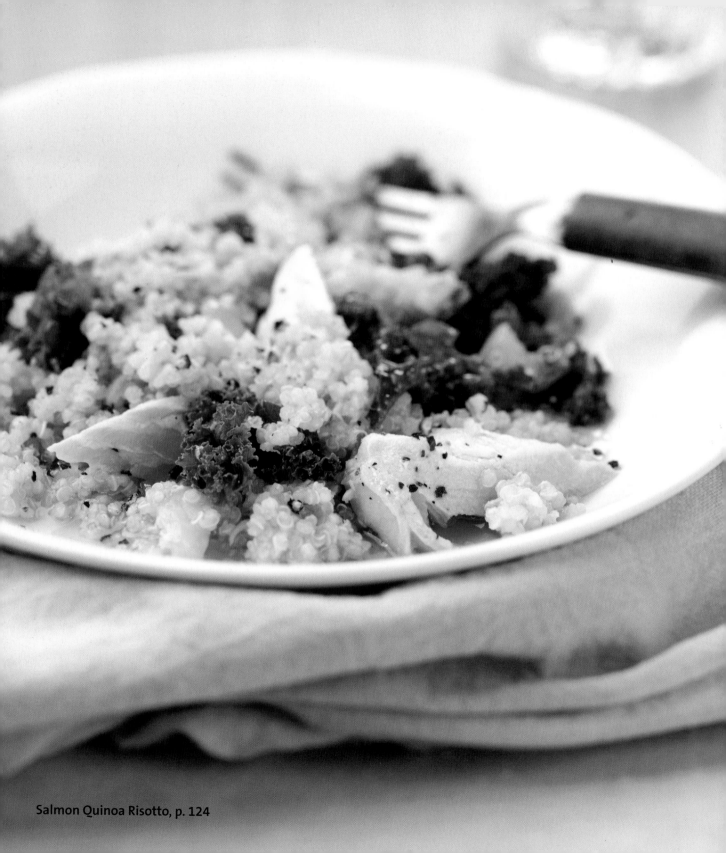

Salmon Quinoa Risotto, p. 124

CHAPTER 6

One Pot and Skillet

Baked Turkey Meatballs | 112

Caramelized Onion Chicken | 113

Cherry Glazed Pork Loin Chops | 114

Chicken with White Wine Garlic Sauce | 115

Costa Rican Black Beans and Rice (Gallo Pinto) | 116

Country Captain Chicken | 117

Grilled Salmon with Sweet Balsamic Onions | 118

Lemon Garlic Shrimp | 119

Potato Crusted Bacon Quiche | 121

Potato Frittata | 122

Red Bean Casserole | 123

Salmon Quinoa Risotto | 124

Shrimp Provençal | 125

Baked Turkey Meatballs*

1/2 teaspoon olive oil

1 pound lean ground turkey

1/2 cup grated carrots

1/2 cup grated onions

1 teaspoon fresh thyme

1 teaspoon lemon zest

1 teaspoon parsley (finely chopped)

1/4 teaspoon ancho chile powder

1/4 cup saltine-type crackers (crushed fine)

1 large egg

1/2 cup white wine

1/2 teaspoon kosher salt

1/4 teaspoon fresh ground pepper

1 tablespoon grated Parmesan cheese (optional)

Everyone loves meatballs. Serve them with whole grain pasta, brown rice, with a side of sautéed broccoli or carrots, or all by themselves. They keep well in the freezer; just thaw them out in the refrigerator and you can have dinner ready in a flash.

1 Preheat oven to 350°F.

2 Use the olive oil to lightly oil an 8 × 8-inch square baking dish.

3 In a large bowl, thoroughly mix all of the remaining ingredients, except for the Parmesan cheese.

4 To form the meatballs, pull a handful (about 1/2 cup) of the turkey mixture and toss back and forth in your hands to form a ball. The ball should form rather easily.

5 Once the meatballs are formed, place them in the baking dish.

6 Cover with foil and bake for 40 minutes. Remove the foil and continue baking for an additional 15 minutes.

7 Remove the meatballs from the oven and sprinkle with Parmesan cheese.

*Recipe courtesy of Pamela Braun

EXCHANGES/ CHOICES		
1/2 Carbohydrate 2 Lean Meat 1/2 Fat	Calories **160** Calories from Fat **70** Total Fat **8.0 g** Saturated Fat **2.0 g** Trans Fat **0.1 g** Cholesterol **95 mg**	Sodium **260 mg** Total Carbohydrate **5 g** · Dietary Fiber **1 g** Sugars **1 g** Protein **17 g**

Caramelized Onion Chicken

1/2 cup no-sugar-added, red raspberry jam

1 1/2 teaspoons fresh grated ginger

1 tablespoon red wine vinegar

1 tablespoon lower-sodium soy sauce

1 pound boneless, skinless, halved chicken breasts, 1/2-inch thick

1/4 teaspoon salt

1/4 teaspoon fresh ground black pepper

1 1/2 tablespoons canola oil, divided

1 medium onion, halved and sliced

Kids just love this recipe. You can also use orange marmalade, peach, or apricot jam for a variety of flavors. For another version, try substituting for the chicken with 1/2-inch thick, boneless pork loin chops.

1   In a small bowl, combine the raspberry jam, ginger, red wine vinegar, and soy sauce, and set aside. Sprinkle the chicken with salt and pepper.

2   Heat 1 tablespoon of oil in a large skillet. Sear the chicken over medium-high heat for about 5 minutes per side. Remove the chicken from the pan and set aside.

3   Heat the remaining 1/2 tablespoon oil in the skillet. Sauté the onion for about 4–5 minutes, until browned. Add the raspberry sauce and lower the heat to simmer for 1–2 minutes. Add the chicken breasts back in and cook for 2 more minutes.

EXCHANGES/ CHOICES		
1 1/2 Carbohydrate	Calories **275**	Sodium **360 mg**
3 Lean Meat	Calories from Fat **70**	Total Carbohydrate **24 g**
1/2 Fat	Total Fat **8.0 g**	Dietary Fiber **1 g**
	Saturated Fat **1.2 g**	Sugars **18 g**
	Trans Fat **0.0 g**	Protein **25 g**
	Cholesterol **65 mg**	

A Bouquet Garni

A Bouquet Garni is a little bundle of herbs and spices tied together in a cheesecloth packet that gives great flavor to one pot meals. Here's how to make a bouquet garni:

Parsley, thyme, and bay leaf are the traditional herbs and spices included in a bouquet garni. One or more of the following can be added to create interesting deep flavor to your food:

• A strip of orange zest enhances one pot meals made with lean beef

• A few cloves for warmth and sweetness

• A sprig of rosemary adds a Mediterranean flavor

• A peeled garlic clove is always a welcomed addition

Add the basic three plus one of the flavor add-ins to a 5 × 5-inch piece of cheesecloth. Gather the four sides of the cheesecloth together and tie the packet with string. I like to place the bouquet garni packet under the meat or vegetables in the bottom of the pan. As it cooks, the flavors are extracted and permeate the dish.

Cherry Glazed Pork Loin Chops

4 (5 ounces each) bone-in pork loin chops (about 3/4-inch thick)

kosher salt, to taste

freshly ground black pepper, to taste

2 teaspoons canola oil

SAUCE

1 small shallot, minced

1 1/2 cups low-fat, reduced-sodium chicken broth

1/2 cup ruby port wine

1/2 cup dried cherries

3 tablespoons fat-free milk

1 1/2 teaspoons cornstarch

2 teaspoons minced fresh thyme

2 teaspoons minced fresh parsley

This is a terrific recipe for the holidays (or easily prepared on a Tuesday night). Serve the chops with a crisp green salad and roasted potatoes.

1   Pat the pork chops dry and sprinkle them on both sides with salt and pepper.

2   Heat the oil in a large 12-inch skillet over medium-high heat. Add the pork chops and sear for about 4–5 minutes per side. Remove the pork chops from the skillet onto a plate. Tent the pork chops with foil and set aside.

3   In the pan drippings, add the shallot and sauté for 1 minute. Add in the broth, port, and cherries. Bring to a simmer and cook until reduced to about 3/4 cup. Scrape up any browned bits.

4   Meanwhile, whisk together the milk and cornstarch. Add the milk-cornstarch mixture to the pan and cook for 1–2 minutes, until thickened. Add back the pork chops and simmer the pork chops in the sauce for 2–3 minutes. Garnish with fresh thyme and parsley.

EXCHANGES/ CHOICES		
1 Fruit	Calories **260**	Sodium **245 mg**
1/2 Carbohydrate	Calories from Fat **70**	Total Carbohydrate **21 g**
3 Lean Meat	Total Fat **8.0 g**	Dietary Fiber **1 g**
1/2 Fat	Saturated Fat **2.3 g**	Sugars **15 g**
	Trans Fat **0.0 g**	Protein **22 g**
	Cholesterol **60 mg**	

Chicken with White Wine Garlic Sauce

3 tablespoons flour, divided

1 1/2 teaspoons dried sage

1 1/2 teaspoons dried rosemary

kosher salt, to taste

freshly ground black pepper, to taste

1 1/2 pounds boneless, skinless chicken thighs or breasts (or combo of both)

2 tablespoons olive oil

20 garlic cloves, peeled and sliced

1/4 teaspoon crushed red pepper flakes

1 onion, chopped

1/2 cup dry white wine

1 1/4 cups low-fat, reduced-sodium chicken broth

1 tablespoon butter

3 tablespoons chopped parsley

No, it's not a typo; there are indeed 20 cloves of garlic in this dish. But don't worry; this dish is completely mellow and very comforting. This is lovely served over cooked noodles, over rice, or just all by itself.

1 Preheat the oven to 325°F. Combine 2 tablespoons of flour, sage, rosemary, salt, and pepper on a plate.

2 Dredge the chicken in the flour mixture and shake off excess.

3 Heat oil in a large skillet over medium-high heat. Add the chicken to the pan and cook for 4 minutes per side. Transfer to a baking sheet and continue to cook in the preheated oven until chicken is cooked through, about 25 minutes.

4 Meanwhile, add the garlic, red pepper flakes, and onion to the pan and cook until garlic begins to brown.

5 Stir in the wine and scrape the browned bits. Add the chicken broth and boil until reduced by half, about 8–10 minutes. Remove from heat.

6 Whisk together the butter and 1 tablespoon flour and add to the pan and whisk well. Return the pan to the heat and cook until the sauce thickens. Pour the sauce over the chicken and sprinkle with parsley.

EXCHANGES/CHOICES		
1 1/2 Starch	Calories **285**	Sodium **145 mg**
1 Vegetable	Calories from Fat **80**	Total Carbohydrate **27 g**
2 Lean Meat	Total Fat **9.0 g**	Dietary Fiber **2 g**
1 Fat	Saturated Fat **2.3 g**	Sugars **1 g**
	Trans Fat **0.1 g**	Protein **23 g**
	Cholesterol **75 mg**	

Costa Rican Black Beans and Rice (Gallo Pinto)*

1 cup white rice

2 tablespoons olive oil

1 green bell pepper, finely diced

1 small yellow onion, finely diced

1 1/2 teaspoons (about 3 cloves) minced garlic

1 teaspoon cumin

1/2 teaspoon curry powder

1 15-ounce can black beans with their liquid

2 tablespoons Worcestershire sauce

2 tablespoons salsa (optional)

1/2 cup fresh cilantro (optional)

1 lime, cut into wedges for serving (optional)

This Costa Rican favorite called Gallo Pinto (which translates as "painted rooster") is served with nearly every meal. It's great comfort food for any season and the curry and lime give it a Caribbean flair. For even more Caribbean flavor, cook the rice in half water and half coconut milk. Serve it with warm tortillas and fresh pineapple (another Costa Rican specialty).

1 Cook the rice with 2 cups of water according to the package directions. (The rice can be made up to a day in advance.)

2 In a large skillet, heat the oil over medium heat and sauté the pepper, onion, and garlic for about 5 minutes until they are fragrant and slightly tender. While they are cooking, stir in the cumin and curry powder. Add the beans and their liquid, the Worcestershire sauce, and salsa (optional) and bring it to a boil.

3 Let the mixture simmer for 5 minutes. Stir in the cooked rice and continue to cook it for about 3 more minutes until it is heated through. Stir in the cilantro, if desired, and serve it with the lime wedges. Serve it immediately or refrigerate it for up to 3 days.

*Recipe courtesy of Aviva Goldfarb

EXCHANGES/ CHOICES		
1/2 Carbohydrate 2 Lean Meat	Calories **130** Calories from Fat **35**	Sodium **210 mg** Total Carbohydrate **6 g**
	Total Fat **4.0 g** Saturated Fat **1.4 g** Trans Fat **0.0 g**	Dietary Fiber **0 g** Sugars **3 g**
	Cholesterol **65 mg**	Protein **16 g**

Country Captain Chicken

2 teaspoons olive oil

4 (5 ounces each) boneless, skinless chicken breast halves

1 small onion, thinly sliced

4 cloves garlic, minced`

1/2 tablespoon curry powder

1 14-ounce can diced tomatoes in juice, undrained

1/4 cup dried apricots, thinly sliced

1/2 tablespoon minced fresh thyme

1 teaspoon paprika

1 teaspoon crushed red pepper

kosher salt, to taste

freshly ground black pepper, to taste

1/4 cup sliced almonds

This is one of those "lost" recipes that was served back in the 50s and 60s. A beautiful mélange of chicken, tomatoes, and intensely flavored dried apricots makes for a perfect one pot dinner.

1   Heat oil in large Dutch oven over medium heat. Add chicken and sauté until golden brown, about 3 minutes per side. With tongs or slotted spoon, transfer chicken to plate.

2   Add onion and garlic to pan and cook until onion is tender, about 5 minutes.

3   Stir in curry powder and cook for 1 minute. Add tomatoes, apricots, thyme, paprika, crushed red pepper, salt, and pepper, and bring to a boil.

4   Return chicken (and any accumulated juices) to Dutch oven. Reduce to a simmer, cover, and cook until chicken is cooked through, about 20 minutes. Meanwhile, toast the almonds in a small, dry skillet over medium heat, until the almonds are golden brown. Garnish the chicken with the almonds.

EXCHANGES/ CHOICES		
1/2 Fruit	Calories **270**	Sodium **220 mg**
1 Vegetable	Calories from Fat **80**	Total Carbohydrate **15 g**
4 Lean Meat	Total Fat **9.0 g**	Dietary Fiber **3 g**
1/2 Fat	Saturated Fat **1.6 g**	Sugars **9 g**
	Trans Fat **0.0 g**	Protein **33 g**
	Cholesterol **80 mg**	

Fast Fixes for Rice

Sometimes rice burns and sometimes it gets too mushy. Here are some tips to prevent both and more.

- If rice is still very chewy or hard after the allotted cooking time, add just enough water to create some steam. Cover and cook on very low heat for 5 minutes.

- If your rice is cooked through but still seems too wet, uncover the pot and cook on low heat for a few minutes more. Or spread the rice on a baking sheet and dry at 250°F.

- If rice completely splits and becomes too mushy, save it and make a rice pudding.

- If the bottom of the rice is burned, run cold water on the outside of the pot's bottom and try to salvage the good rice.

Grilled Salmon With Sweet Balsamic Onions

ONIONS

2 teaspoons olive oil

1 large sweet onion, halved and sliced thin

2 tablespoons balsamic vinegar

1/4 teaspoon dried thyme leaves

1/2 cup water

2 teaspoons sugar

SALMON

4 (4 ounces each) salmon filets

1 tablespoon all-purpose flour

1/2 teaspoon kosher salt

1/4 teaspoon freshly ground black pepper

1 teaspoon olive oil

There is absolutely nothing I like better than caramelized onions smothered over a simply prepared piece of meat, poultry, or fish. This one pot grilled salmon dish is blanketed under a glorious mound of sweet onions. Use the onion preparation part of the recipe and add to cooked vegetables too.

1   Heat the olive oil in a medium skillet over medium heat. Add the onions and sauté for 2 minutes. Add the balsamic vinegar and thyme and sauté for 5 minutes. Add the water and sugar and continue to sauté until the onions absorb the water, about 8–12 minutes. Add more water if necessary.

2   Combine the flour, salt, and pepper. Dredge the salmon lightly in the flour mixture. Heat the oil in a large skillet over medium-high heat.

3   Sear the salmon on medium-high heat for about 3–4 minutes per side or until desired doneness.

4   Serve the salmon smothered with the onions.

EXCHANGES/ CHOICES		
1 Carbohydrate 4 Lean Meat 1 Fat	Calories **280** Calories from Fat **125** Total Fat **14.0 g** Saturated Fat **2.2 g** Trans Fat **0.0 g** Cholesterol **80 mg**	Sodium **310 mg** Total Carbohydrate **11 g** Dietary Fiber **1 g** Sugars **7 g** Protein **26 g**

Lemon Garlic Shrimp

4 garlic cloves, minced

1/4 teaspoon crushed red pepper flakes

2 tablespoons olive oil

1 pound peeled and deveined large shrimp

1/2 cup dry white wine

1 tablespoon lemon juice

1/2 cup low-fat, reduced-sodium chicken broth

1/2 teaspoon grated lemon zest

1/4 teaspoon kosher salt

1/4 teaspoon freshly ground black pepper

Very much like the classic shrimp scampi, but with a whole lot less fat. The fresh lemon and lemon zest really carry the flavors. These ingredients should be part of your pantry staples, so this meal can come together quickly in under 30 minutes.

1   Heat the oil in a large skillet over medium heat. Add the garlic and crushed red pepper and sauté for 30 seconds. Add the shrimp and sauté for 3–4 minutes, until shrimp is cooked through and turns pink. Remove the shrimp from the skillet.

2   Add the wine and lemon juice and bring to a boil. Add the broth and bring back to a boil. Season with lemon zest, salt, and pepper. Pour over the shrimp and serve.

EXCHANGES/ CHOICES

4 Lean Meat
1/2 Fat

Calories **195**
Calories from Fat **70**
Total Fat **8.0 g**
Saturated Fat **1.2 g**
Trans Fat **0.0 g**
Cholesterol **185 mg**

Sodium **355 mg**
Total Carbohydrate **2 g**
Dietary Fiber **0 g**
Sugars **0 g**
Protein **25 g**

Stocking Up

Quick one pot meals call for ingredients for you to have on hand, always! Here is a list of the things that will help you create a one pot meal in a jiffy.

CANNED FISH

Keep cans of water-packed tuna, salmon, and sardines on hand for tossing into hot and cold one pot meals.

GRAINS

The fast cooking ones include bulgur wheat, couscous, polenta, and quinoa.

LENTILS AND CANNED BEANS

Lentils never need soaking, just cook them up fast, often in less than 20 minutes. Canned beans have to be one of the most convenient sources of "fast food" around! Just remember to rinse them in a colander with cold water to get rid of some of the sodium.

CANNED TOMATOES

Buy them whole, diced, and crushed. Great for a variety of one pot meals.

BOTTLED SAUCES

Keep low-sodium soy sauce, oyster, chili, and hoisin sauces as well as mustard, Worcestershire sauce, and Tabasco sauce in your kitchen.

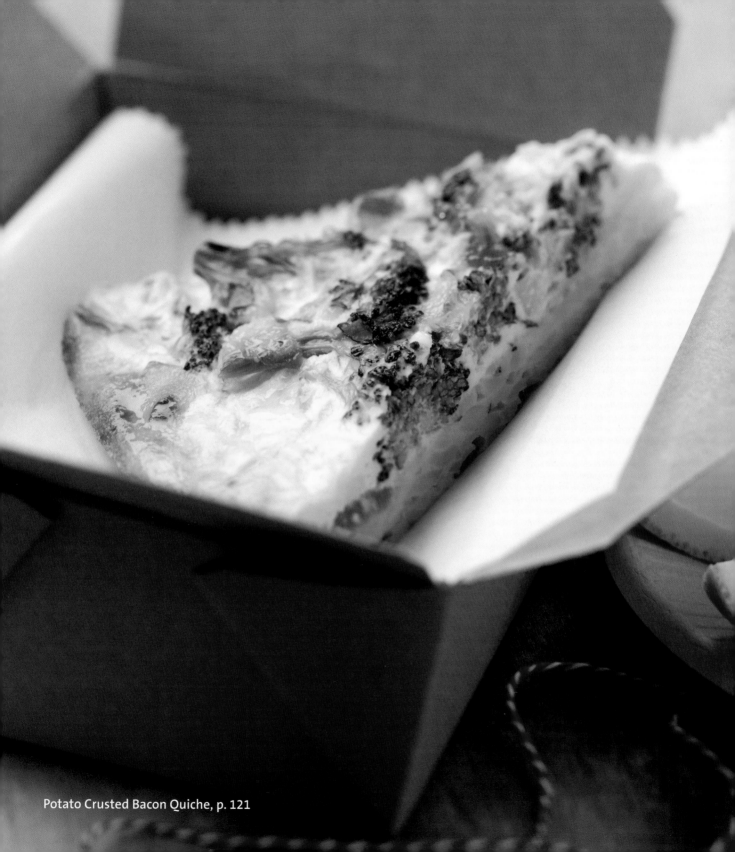

Potato Crusted Bacon Quiche, p. 121

Potato Crusted Bacon Quiche

CRUST

2 1/2 cups frozen, shredded hash browns, thawed, with excess water drained

1 egg white, beaten until frothy

1 tablespoon Parmesan cheese

1 teaspoon dried basil

1/4 teaspoon kosher salt

FILLING

2 slices reduced-fat bacon

1 small onion, chopped

1 10-ounce package frozen chopped broccoli, thawed and drained, patted dry

1 cup 1% milk

1/4 cup fat-free cream cheese

1/4 cup reduced-fat cream cheese

2 eggs

2 egg whites

2 tablespoons chopped fresh parsley

1/2 teaspoon kosher salt

1/4 teaspoon freshly ground black pepper

1/2 cup extra-sharp reduced-fat cheddar cheese (such as 75% less fat Cabot extra sharp cheddar)

Quiche is the ultimate comfort food. But this time, we eliminate the fatty pastry crust in favor of something much more fun!! By using frozen shredded hash browns, we eliminate the fat and add some crispy crunchy texture that adds a double dose of comfort to a true favorite.

1   Preheat the oven to 425°F. To make the crust, combine the crust ingredients and press into a 9-inch quiche or pie pan, covering the sides and bottom. Bake the crust for 10 minutes and remove from the oven and set aside.

2   Cook the bacon in a large skillet over medium-high heat until crispy, about 3 minutes. Remove from the skillet and crumble. In the pan drippings sauté the onion, add the frozen thawed broccoli, and sauté for 3 minutes.

3   In a bowl, combine the milk, cream cheeses, eggs, egg whites, parsley, salt, and pepper. Mix well. Add the cheddar cheese and cooked bacon.

4   Spread the broccoli mixture on the bottom of the cooked crust. Pour over the milk mixture. Bake for 15 minutes at 425°F. Lower the heat to 325°F and continue to cook for about 35 minutes until a knife inserted comes out clean.

EXCHANGES/ CHOICES		
1/2 Carbohydrate 1 Med-Fat Meat	Calories **120** Calories from Fat **40** Total Fat **4.5 g** Saturated Fat **2.2 g** Trans Fat **0.0 g** Cholesterol **65 mg**	Sodium **405 mg** Total Carbohydrate **10 g** Dietary Fiber **2 g** Sugars **3 g** Protein **10 g**

Potato Frittata

1/4 cup fat-free milk

4 eggs

4 egg whites

sea salt, to taste

freshly ground black
  pepper, to taste

2 teaspoons olive oil

1 large onion, diced

1/2 pound small red-
  skinned potatoes, thinly
  sliced

1/4 cup low-fat, reduced-
  sodium chicken broth

1 1/2 tablespoons freshly
  grated Parmesan cheese

2 tablespoons minced
  fresh chives

Scrambled eggs might be quicker to prepare, but I consider frittatas much more comforting. The opportunity to cram as many fillings you want into this pancake-like concoction is always a great culinary challenge.

1   In a large bowl, whisk together the milk, eggs, egg whites, salt, and pepper. Set aside.

2   Heat the olive oil in a 10-inch nonstick ovenproof skillet over medium heat. Add the onion and sauté for 5 minutes. Add the potatoes and sauté for 5 minutes. Add the broth, cover, and cook over medium heat until potatoes are browned, and broth is absorbed, about 8 minutes.

3   Pour the egg mixture over the potatoes, cover and cook on low heat for about 10–12 minutes until almost set. Preheat the oven broiler.

4   Sprinkle the frittata with the cheese. Transfer the skillet to the oven and broil about 6 inches from the heat source until cheese is melted and is lightly browned, about 3 minutes. Sprinkle the frittata with fresh chives and cut into wedges to serve.

EXCHANGES/ CHOICES		
1/2 Starch	Calories **125**	Sodium **125 mg**
1 Lean Meat	Calories from Fat **45**	Total Carbohydrate **11 g**
1 Fat	Total Fat **5.0 g**	Dietary Fiber **1 g**
	Saturated Fat **1.5 g**	Sugars **3 g**
	Trans Fat **0.0 g**	Protein **9 g**
	Cholesterol **140 mg**	

Red Bean Casserole

3/4 pound boneless, skinless chicken breasts, cubed into 1-inch pieces

4 garlic cloves, finely minced

1/2 teaspoon dried thyme

kosher salt, to taste

freshly ground black pepper, to taste

1 1/2 tablespoons olive oil, divided

1 large onion, chopped

2 medium carrots, peeled and julienned

1 cup canned whole tomatoes, coarsely chopped, with their juice

1/4 cup dry white wine

1 can kidney beans, drained and rinsed (about 3 cups)

3/4 teaspoon fresh orange zest

4 tablespoons plain dry breadcrumbs*

The secret to this casserole is in the orange zest. It provides a clean, fresh taste to this one pot casserole. This is somewhat like cassoulet, but because it contains no red meat, it's so much better for you. The red beans provide more of the protein with the added bonus of good fiber.

1 Toss the chicken cubes with the garlic, thyme, salt, and pepper in a small bowl. Cover and refrigerate for 1 hour.

2 In a Dutch oven or similar pot, heat 1 tablespoon of the olive oil over medium heat. Add the chicken and sauté for 4–5 minutes. Transfer the chicken to a plate.

3 Preheat the oven to 400°F. Add the onion and carrots to the pan and sauté for about 6–7 minutes until the onion is soft. Add the tomatoes with juice, wine, beans, and orange zest. Bring to a boil. Lower the heat and add chicken to the pan. Cover, transfer pot to the oven, and bake for 20 minutes.

4 Combine 1/2 tablespoon of olive oil and the breadcrumbs. Uncover the pot and sprinkle the breadcrumbs on top of the casserole. Bake for another 10 minutes, until the crumbs are browned.

* Fresh breadcrumbs may be used. Use stale bread, preferably Italian bread, and process in a food processor or blender to make coarse crumbs.

EXCHANGES/ CHOICES		
2 Starch 1 Vegetable 3 Lean Meat	Calories **310** Calories from Fat **65** Total Fat **7.0 g** Saturated Fat **1.2 g** Trans Fat **0.0 g** Cholesterol **40 mg**	Sodium **335 mg** Total Carbohydrate **37 g** Dietary Fiber **9 g** Sugars **5 g** Protein **25 g**

Salmon Quinoa Risotto*

1 1/2 tablespoons olive oil, divided

1 medium onion, diced

1 cup quinoa

4 cups organic vegetable stock, divided

4–5 garlic cloves, finely chopped

7–8 leaves of kale, stems removed and cut into ribbons

10 ounces salmon, poached and flaked

salt, to taste

pepper, to taste

Quinoa is not the usual grain in risotto, but this protein-packed, tiny grain cooks quickly and results in a wonderfully fragrant risotto-like dish.

1 To poach salmon—Fill a 4-quart saucepan with water and put salmon filet into the water. Place saucepan over high heat until water boils. Once water boils, remove pan from heat and let sit for 10 minutes. Remove fish from water and flake. Set aside.

2 In a 4-quart saucepan, heat 1 tablespoon of olive oil over medium-high heat. When oil is shimmering, add diced onion. Sauté onion until transparent. Add quinoa to onion mixture and stir—to toast—for 2 minutes.

3 Add 1 cup of vegetable stock to quinoa and onion. Stir until stock is absorbed. Once stock is absorbed, add another 1 cup of stock. Continue stirring until stock is absorbed. Add remaining stock in 1/2-cup intervals, stirring until all stock is absorbed. Remove from heat.

4 While preparing the onion quinoa mixture, heat 1/2 tablespoon of oil over medium-high heat in a sauté pan with chopped garlic. Once garlic is sizzling, add chopped kale to the pan. Turn kale to coat with oil and garlic. Turn kale mixture until fragrant, approximately 2 minutes. Remove kale mixture from heat.

5 Once quinoa is complete, add kale and salmon. Stir to combine and add salt and pepper to taste.

EXCHANGES/ CHOICES

2 Starch
1 Vegetable
3 Lean Meat
1 1/2 Fat

Calories **390**
 Calories from Fat **115**

Total Fat **13.0 g**
 Saturated Fat **2.2 g**
 Trans Fat **0.0 g**

Cholesterol **40 mg**

Sodium **195 mg**

Total Carbohydrate **39 g**
 Dietary Fiber **5 g**
 Sugars **5 g**

Protein **27 g**

*Recipe courtesy of Pamela Braun

Shrimp Provençal

1 tablespoon canola oil

1 onion, diced

2 cloves garlic

3 tablespoons white wine

1 pound large peeled and deveined shrimp

2 tablespoons minced parsley

1/2 teaspoon dried oregano

1 14 1/2-ounce can diced tomatoes

1 tablespoon balsamic vinegar

1/4 cup halved black olives

2 teaspoons drained capers

dash hot sauce

1/4 cup basil chiffonade (thinly sliced basil)

When I first traveled to Italy, I was actually surprised to learn that the best cooks use everyday pantry items. We typically think that Italian cooks use only fresh ingredients, and they mostly do, but they also use lots of shelf staple ingredients like the canned tomatoes in this flavorful recipe.

1   Heat the oil in a large skillet over medium-high heat. Add the onion and garlic and sauté for 2–3 minutes. Add the wine and let simmer until reduced. Add the shrimp and flip over after 2 minutes.

2   Add the parsley, oregano, tomatoes, vinegar, olives, capers, and hot sauce. Bring to a simmer for 3 minutes, or until shrimp are fully cooked.

3   Serve with a sprinkle of basil chiffonade.

EXCHANGES/ CHOICES		
2 Vegetable 3 Lean Meat	Calories **200** Calories from Fat **55** Total Fat **6.0 g** Saturated Fat **0.7 g** Trans Fat **0.0 g** Cholesterol **185 mg**	Sodium **435 mg** Total Carbohydrate **10 g** Dietary Fiber **2 g** Sugars **5 g** Protein **26 g**

One Pot Meals with Rice, Grains, and Beans

Toss cooked rice, grains, or beans with a small amount of olive oil. Add sliced, rehydrated sun-dried tomatoes, a can of flaked salmon, and some chopped fresh basil and parsley.

Mix cooked beans, rice, or other grains with a jar of your favorite salsa. Add diced, fresh tomatoes, a small amount of diced avocado, and sprinkle with lemon juice.

Mix cooked rice or other grains with a can of low-fat chili, 2 tablespoons shredded low-fat cheese and warm in the microwave. Top with a dollop of plain, nonfat yogurt and chopped scallions.

Penne with Broccoli Rabe, Prosciutto, and Garlic, p. 131

CHAPTER 7
Pasta

Baked Ziti | 128

Chicken and Noodle Salad with Peanut Dressing | 129

Pasta Primavera | 130

Penne with Broccoli Rabe, Prosciutto, and Garlic | 131

Really Quick Pancetta Penne | 132

Rigatoni with Sausage | 133

Spaghetti Agli Olio | 134

Shrimp and Pasta Bowl with Feta | 135

Spaghetti Bolognese | 136

Spaghetti Carbonara | 137

Straw and Hay | 138

Stuffed Shells Florentine | 140

Tagliatelle with Creamy Goat Cheese Sauce | 141

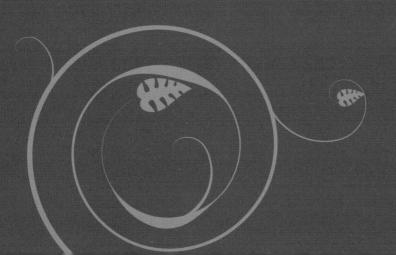

Baked Ziti

8 ounces ziti

2 teaspoons olive oil

4 ounces reduced-fat Italian sausage, casing removed

1/2 cup chopped onion

2 cups bottled marinara sauce

1 cup part-skim mozzarella cheese

2 tablespoons grated fresh Parmesan cheese

GARNISH

1/4 cup minced fresh parsley

This dish is soooo good! Go ahead and try it out on your friends and family. I bet you'll have the whole table saying "Grazie!!"

1 Preheat the oven to 350°F. Coat a 3-quart casserole dish with cooking spray. Set aside.

2 Cook the ziti in a large pot of boiling water according to package directions.

3 Meanwhile, heat the olive oil in a large skillet over medium heat. Sauté the sausage and onion for about 5–7 minutes, breaking up the pieces of sausage.

4 Drain the ziti and add to a large bowl. Add the sausage onion mixture, marinara sauce, and 1 cup of the mozzarella cheese. Spoon into the prepared baking dish.

5 Cover with foil and bake for 40 minutes. Uncover and sprinkle with the remaining mozzarella cheese and Parmesan cheese. Bake for 5–10 minutes until cheese is melted. Sprinkle each serving with fresh parsley.

EXCHANGES/ CHOICES		
1 1/2 Starch 1 Med-Fat Meat	Calories **190** Calories from Fat **55**	Sodium **455 mg** Total Carbohydrate **25 g**
	Total Fat **6.0 g** Saturated Fat **2.5 g** Trans Fat **0.0 g**	Dietary Fiber **2 g** Sugars **5 g**
	Cholesterol **15 mg**	Protein **10 g**

Chicken and Noodle Salad with Peanut Dressing

1 pound boneless, skinless chicken breasts

2 large carrots, peeled and grated

1 red bell pepper, diced

2 scallions, thinly sliced on a diagonal

8 ounces udon or soba noodles or whole-wheat linguine

DRESSING

3 tablespoons reduced-fat peanut butter

3 tablespoons lower-sodium soy sauce

1 1/2 tablespoons rice vinegar

2 teaspoons sesame oil

1 teaspoon sugar

1/2 teaspoon grated fresh ginger

1 garlic clove, finely minced to a paste

GARNISH

1/4 cup coarsely chopped toasted cashews

1/4 cup minced fresh cilantro

Noodles in peanut sauce is a take-out favorite, but making your own is quick, healthier, and not difficult to replicate. Using soba, udon, or whole-wheat pasta makes this dish a bit more nutritious than plain white pasta. Use the peanut sauce on cooked vegetables as well.

1   Place the chicken breasts in a large skillet. Cover with water and bring to a gentle boil. Lower the heat, cover, and let simmer for 10 minutes until the chicken is cooked through. Remove the chicken with a slotted spoon and let it cool on a plate in the refrigerator for 15–20 minutes.

2   Meanwhile, bring a large pot of water to a boil. Combine the carrots, red pepper, and scallions in a large salad bowl.

3   Add the noodles to the boiling water and cook according to package directions. Drain.

4   Combine all the dressing ingredients and mix well. Set aside.

5   Slice the cooled chicken into thin strips and add to the vegetables in the bowl. Add the pasta and the peanut dressing to the bowl and mix well. Garnish the salad with cashews and cilantro.

EXCHANGES/ CHOICES		
1 Starch	Calories **205**	Sodium **300 mg**
1/2 Carbohydrate	Calories from Fat **65**	Total Carbohydrate **21 g**
2 Lean Meat	Total Fat **7.0 g**	Dietary Fiber **2 g**
	Saturated Fat **1.4 g**	Sugars **4 g**
	Trans Fat **0.0 g**	Protein **16 g**
	Cholesterol **25 mg**	

Pasta Primavera

12 ounces penne or other pasta shapes

1/2 pound asparagus, cut into 1 1/2-inch lengths (keep tips separate)

1/2 pound green beans, trimmed and cut into 1/4-inch lengths

1/2 pound shelled fresh peas

1 tablespoon olive oil

1 onion, chopped

1 garlic clove, chopped

3 ounces lean pancetta, chopped

1/4 pound button mushrooms, chopped

1 tablespoon flour

3/4 cup dry white wine

2 tablespoons half-and-half

2 tablespoons chopped mixed fresh herbs, such as parsley and thyme

kosher salt, to taste

freshly ground black pepper, to taste

Pasta Primavera literally translates to springtime pasta. We typically associate comfort food with a cold winter night, but this is great when the spring flowers begin to bloom. The sauce is light, yet creamy, so it's comforting without all the usual heaviness.

1 Cook the pasta in boiling water for 10–12 minutes, or according to the package instructions. Drain well.

2 While the pasta is cooking, drop the pieces of asparagus stalk, green beans, and peas into a saucepan of boiling water. Bring back to a boil and cook for 5 minutes. Add the asparagus tips and cook for 2 minutes. Drain thoroughly.

3 Heat the oil in a saucepan. Add the onion and cook for 3–4 minutes or until softened. Add the garlic, pancetta, and mushrooms, and continue to cook, stirring occasionally, for about 2 minutes.

4 Stir in the flour, then gradually pour in the wine and bring to the boil, stirring constantly. Simmer until the sauce is thickened. Stir in the half-and-half, herbs, and season with the salt and pepper. Add the vegetables to the sauce and heat gently for 1–2 minutes, without boiling.

5 Divide the pasta among 4 serving bowls and spoon the sauce over the top. Serve immediately.

EXCHANGES/ CHOICES		
3 Starch	Calories **355**	Sodium **275 mg**
1 Vegetable	Calories from Fat **80**	Total Carbohydrate **55 g**
2 Fat	Total Fat **9.0 g**	Dietary Fiber **6 g**
	Saturated Fat **2.4 g**	Sugars **6 g**
	Trans Fat **0.0 g**	Protein **14 g**
	Cholesterol **15 mg**	

Penne with Broccoli Rabe, Prosciutto, and Garlic

8 ounces uncooked penne pasta

1 tablespoon olive oil

4 garlic cloves, minced

1/2 teaspoon crushed red pepper

2 cups broccoli rabe, trimmed and cut into 2-inch pieces

1/2 cup sliced sun-dried tomatoes

1/2 cup water

2 tablespoons freshly grated Parmesan cheese

1/2 cup fat-free ricotta cheese

1/3 cup soft, reduced-fat goat cheese

2 slices prosciutto di Parma, sliced 1/8-inch thick and diced

2 tablespoons minced parsley

kosher salt, to taste

freshly ground black pepper, to taste

Broccoli rabe, a cousin of broccoli, is considered a homey comfort food among the Italians. Sun-dried tomatoes and lots of garlic add so much to this fast, easy dish.

1   Bring a pot of water to boil for the pasta. Add the pasta and cook for 10 minutes.

2   In a sauté pan, add the olive oil and bring to medium-high heat.

3   Add garlic, red pepper, broccoli rabe, sun-dried tomatoes, and 1/2 cup water and cook covered with a lid for 5 minutes.

4   In a large bowl, add Parmesan cheese, ricotta cheese, goat cheese, and prosciutto and mix gently. Drain the pasta and add it to the bowl. Toss with garlic, broccoli rabe, and sun-dried tomato mixture.

5   Add parsley, salt, and pepper.

EXCHANGES/ CHOICES		
2 Starch 1 Med-Fat Meat	Calories **225** Calories from Fat **45**	Sodium **255 mg** Total Carbohydrate **33 g**
	Total Fat **5.0 g** Saturated Fat **1.7 g** Trans Fat **0.0 g**	Dietary Fiber **2 g** Sugars **4 g**
	Cholesterol **10 mg**	Protein **12 g**

Really Quick Pancetta Penne

8 ounces uncooked penne
noodles

2 ounces pancetta bacon,
chopped

1 medium onion, chopped

1 clove garlic, minced

2 cups bottled marinara
sauce

1/4 cup pitted, chopped
black olives (preferably
Kalamata)

1 tablespoon capers,
drained

2 tablespoons freshly
grated Parmesan cheese

Don't be fooled into thinking that Italians always make
pasta sauces from scratch; they do a little honest cheating
too! In this recipe, good quality bottled sauce is combined
with fabulous, rich-tasting ingredients that make it taste
homemade.

1 Boil the pasta according to package directions, until
cooked al dente, about 7–9 minutes.

2 While the pasta is cooking, sauté the pancetta, onion,
and garlic in a large skillet for 6–7 minutes over
medium-high heat. Add the marinara sauce and cook for
5 minutes.

3 Add the olives and capers. Drain the pasta and
immediately add it to the sauce. Toss well and serve with
Parmesan cheese.

EXCHANGES/ CHOICES		
3 1/2 Starch	Calories **360**	Sodium **930 mg**
1 Vegetable	Calories from Fat **80**	Total Carbohydrate **58 g**
1 1/2 Fat	Total Fat **9.0 g**	Dietary Fiber **4 g**
	Saturated Fat **2.7 g**	Sugars **14 g**
	Trans Fat **0.0 g**	Protein **13 g**
	Cholesterol **15 mg**	

White, Red, or Green?

Which sauce for which pasta? To Italians, the
sauce should coat the pasta lightly without
leaving a pool on the plate when the pasta has
been eaten. There are no hard and fast rules as
to what type of sauce to serve with what pasta,
but here are a few suggestions:

• Long, thin strands go well
with simple sauces such
as olive oil–based sauces
like pesto. You want just
enough sauce to keep the
strands separate.

• Thicker strands go well with
a creamy sauce or a smooth
tomato sauce.

• Shaped pasta goes well
with chunkier vegetable
sauces.

Rigatoni with Sausage

8 ounces rigatoni

1 teaspoon olive oil

3 ounces hot Italian sausage, casings removed

1 large onion, chopped

4 garlic cloves, minced

1 small zucchini, diced

1 14 1/2-ounce can diced tomatoes

3 tablespoons chopped fresh basil

2 teaspoons chopped fresh oregano

1/4 cup pitted black olives

GARNISH

1/4 cup chopped fresh parsley

Rigatoni with sausage was a staple in my home growing up. My mom always seemed to have the ingredients on hand, and over the years she continued to slim it down. This is the version I remember so well because it filled me up, but never weighed me down.

1 Boil the pasta in a large pot of lightly salted water for about 10–12 minutes or until al dente. Drain, set aside.

2 Heat the oil in a large skillet over medium heat. Add the sausage and onion and cook for 3 minutes, making sure to break apart the sausage.

3 Add the garlic and cook for 2 minutes. Add in the zucchini and cook for 4 minutes.

4 Add in the tomatoes (with juice) and bring to a boil. Lower the heat, cover, and simmer for 15 minutes. Add in the basil, oregano, and olives and cook uncovered for 3 minutes.

5 Toss in the pasta and mix well. Serve in a shallow bowl and garnish with chopped parsley.

EXCHANGES/ CHOICES		
1 1/2 Starch 1 Vegetable 1/2 Fat	Calories **165** Calories from Fat **30** Total Fat **3.5 g** Saturated Fat **0.9 g** Trans Fat **0.0 g** Cholesterol **5 mg**	Sodium **195 mg** Total Carbohydrate **27 g** Dietary Fiber **2 g** Sugars **4 g** Protein **6 g**

Spaghetti Agli Olio

8 ounces uncooked spaghetti (you may use any shaped pasta)

4 tablespoons olive oil

6 garlic cloves, thinly sliced

1/4 to 1/2 teaspoon crushed red pepper (depending on your tolerance for hot pepper)

1 1/2 cups fresh baby spinach leaves

1/4 cup freshly grated Parmesan cheese

1/4 teaspoon freshly ground black pepper

By looking at the short ingredient list, you might not think this dish would amount to tasting like anything great. This dish is nothing short of spectacular simplicity.

1   Cook pasta according to package directions.

2   Meanwhile, heat the oil in a large skillet over medium heat. Add the garlic and crushed red pepper and sauté until garlic is slightly browned, about 1 minute.

3   Reserve 2 tablespoons of the cooking water and drain the pasta well. (Make sure there is as little water as possible clinging to the pasta.) Add pasta to the pan with the garlic and red pepper and toss well. Add the spinach and continue to cook until spinach wilts. Add the reserved cooking water and continue to cook 1 more minute.

4   Serve pasta with Parmesan cheese and black pepper sprinkled on top.

EXCHANGES/ CHOICES		
1 1/2 Starch 1 1/2 Fat	Calories **185** Calories from Fat **70** Total Fat **8.0 g** Saturated Fat **1.5 g** Trans Fat **0.0 g** Cholesterol **5 mg**	Sodium **35 mg** Total Carbohydrate **23 g** Dietary Fiber **1 g** Sugars **1 g** Protein **5 g**

Shrimp and Pasta Bowl with Feta*

3 pints cherry tomatoes, sliced in half

3 tablespoons olive oil

kosher salt, to taste

freshly ground black pepper, to taste

3 tablespoons minced garlic

1 1/2 pounds medium shrimp, peeled and deveined

1/2 cup fresh chopped parsley

2 tablespoons fresh lemon juice

2/3 cup crumbled feta cheese

1 16-ounce box whole-wheat penne or fusilli

Perfect for a young family, there are always clean plates when this dish is served. It's so simple to make—you can even teach the kids how to peel and devein the shrimp.

1 Preheat the oven to 450°F. Add the cherry tomatoes to a large 9 × 13-inch baking pan. Pour the olive oil over the tomatoes and sprinkle with salt and pepper. Roast in the oven for about 10 minutes.

2 Add the garlic and roast for approximately 10 minutes more. Remove the baking dish from the oven and stir in the shrimp, parsley, and lemon juice. Sprinkle with the feta.

3 Place the baking dish back into the oven and bake for another 10–12 minutes until shrimp are completely cooked through. Meanwhile, bring a large pot of lightly salted water to a boil. Add in the penne and cook until al dente, about 8–9 minutes. Drain the pasta and place into a large serving bowl. Add in the shrimp mixture and lightly toss. Serve immediately.

*Recipe courtesy of Elisa Zied, RD

EXCHANGES/ CHOICES

3 Starch
1 Vegetable
2 Lean Meat
1 Fat

Calories **385**
  Calories from Fat **90**

Total Fat **10.0 g**
  Saturated Fat **2.9 g**
  Trans Fat **0.1 g**

Cholesterol **120 mg**

Sodium **260 mg**

Total Carbohydrate **51 g**
  Dietary Fiber **8 g**
  Sugars **5 g**

Protein **25 g**

Spaghetti Bolognese

1 tablespoon olive oil

1 large onion, diced

1 carrot, peeled and diced

2 celery stalks, diced

2 garlic cloves, minced

20 rehydrated sun-dried
tomato halves, diced

6 ounces 93% lean ground
beef

3 ounces chicken livers,
chopped

1 28-ounce can whole
tomatoes

1 cup dry red wine

1/2 cup low-fat, reduced-
sodium beef broth

10 ounces whole-wheat
spaghetti

2 teaspoons minced fresh
thyme

3 tablespoons minced
fresh parsley

kosher salt, to taste

freshly ground black
pepper, to taste

Although this is one of my longer cooking sauces, it's definitely worth the wait. This is Italy's finest dish and is the epitome of classic home cooking. As the sauce simmers, you can just absorb the heady fragrance.

1 Heat the olive oil in a large skillet over medium heat. Add the onion, carrot, celery, garlic, and sun-dried tomatoes and sauté 10 minutes until the vegetables are lightly browned.

2 Add in the beef and chicken livers and cook until the meat is browned, about 5 minutes.

3 Add the whole tomatoes to a bowl. With your hands, coarsely chop the tomatoes. Add the tomatoes and the liquid, wine, and beef broth to the pan. Bring to a boil. Lower the heat, cover, and simmer for 30–35 minutes, stirring occasionally.

4 Bring a pot of lightly salted water to a boil. Cook the spaghetti for about 10 minutes until al dente.

5 Meanwhile, add the thyme and parsley to the sauce and cook uncovered on medium-low heat for 10 minutes. Drain the pasta.

6 Mix the spaghetti and meat sauce together until the strands are well coated. Add salt and pepper.

EXCHANGES/ CHOICES		
2 Starch	Calories **255**	Sodium **335 mg**
1 Vegetable	Calories from Fat **45**	Total Carbohydrate **38 g**
1 Lean Meat	Total Fat **5.0 g**	Dietary Fiber **7 g**
1/2 Fat	Saturated Fat **1.2 g**	Sugars **8 g**
	Trans Fat **0.1 g**	Protein **15 g**
	Cholesterol **75 mg**	

Spaghetti Carbonara

8 ounces spaghetti (whole-wheat if desired)

2 ounces serrano ham (if you can't get serrano ham, use a good lean ham)

2 eggs

2 tablespoons light cream

2 tablespoons fat-free half-and-half

1 large garlic clove, minced

2 tablespoons part-skim ricotta cheese

2 tablespoons fat-free ricotta cheese

3 tablespoons freshly grated Parmesan cheese, divided

kosher salt, to taste

freshly ground black pepper, to taste

Yes, Spaghetti Carbonara can be prepared lower in fat. I use the same ingredients as a traditional recipe for carbonara, but I use less of each ingredient and this dish still comes out creamy and comforting.

1 Cook the spaghetti in lightly salted water for about 7–9 minutes until al dente.

2 Meanwhile, add the ham to a dry skillet and cook over high heat for 2–3 minutes until crispy. Remove the ham from the skillet, drain on paper towels, and tear the ham into pieces. Set aside.

3 In a medium-sized bowl, beat the eggs with the cream and half-and-half. Add the garlic, ricotta, and half of the Parmesan cheese. Season with salt and pepper.

4 Drain the pasta. Return the empty pan to the heat and pour in the egg mixture. Heat for 1 minute over low heat, stirring constantly. Add the spaghetti to the pot. Toss the spaghetti with the egg mixture, working quickly to coat the strands with the mixture. Add the ham pieces and toss again. Serve immediately with the remaining Parmesan cheese.

EXCHANGES/ CHOICES		
2 1/2 Starch 1 Med-Fat Meat	Calories **255** Calories from Fat **55** Total Fat **6.0 g** Saturated Fat **2.5 g** Trans Fat **0.0 g** Cholesterol **100 mg**	Sodium **225 mg** Total Carbohydrate **36 g** Dietary Fiber **1 g** Sugars **2 g** Protein **14 g**

Straw and Hay

4 ounces uncooked
  fettuccine

4 ounces uncooked
  spinach fettuccine

1 1/2 teaspoons unsalted
  butter

2 teaspoons minced garlic

1/3 cup half-and-half

1/3 cup fat-free half-and-
  half

1/2 10-ounce package
  frozen peas, thawed

1 tablespoon freshly
  grated Parmesan cheese

kosher salt, to taste

1/4 teaspoon fresh,
  ground black pepper

4 ounces lean cooked ham,
  cut into thin slices

I've always loved to combine two colors of pasta together in a dish. It's fun and it makes the dish look so visually appealing. I've brought down the fat quite a bit, but this dish is still amazingly creamy and filling. The strips of ham and peas add texture and dimension to this very homey meal.

1 In a large pot of boiling water, cook the fettuccine according to package directions.

2 Meanwhile, melt the butter in a large nonstick skillet over medium-low heat. Add the garlic and sauté for 1 minute. Stir in the half-and-half, peas, Parmesan, salt, and pepper. Bring the sauce to simmer and cook for 4 minutes.

3 With a slotted spoon, transfer the pasta directly from the pot to the skillet. Add the ham to the skillet. Turn off the heat and toss the pasta so it absorbs the sauce.

EXCHANGES/ CHOICES		
1 1/2 Starch 1 Lean Meat	Calories **155** Calories from Fat **25** Total Fat **3.0 g** Saturated Fat **1.5 g** Trans Fat **0.0 g** Cholesterol **10 mg**	Sodium **130 mg** Total Carbohydrate **24 g** Dietary Fiber **2 g** Sugars **2 g** Protein **8 g**

Straw and Hay, p. 138

Stuffed Shells Florentine

2 cups bottled marinara sauce

16 jumbo pasta shells

1 1/2 cups fat-free ricotta cheese

1 10-ounce package frozen chopped spinach, thawed and squeezed dry

1/4 cup freshly grated Parmesan cheese

1 egg, beaten

1/4 cup minced fresh basil

dash ground nutmeg

1/2 cup shredded part-skim mozzarella cheese

I have wonderful memories of stuffing pasta shells for weekend dinners when I was a kid. In fact, preparing this dish with my mom is one of the reasons that I grew to love cooking.

1 Preheat the oven to 350°F. Spread the bottom of a 9 × 13-inch pan with 1 cup of the marinara sauce. Set aside.

2 Cook the pasta according to package directions. Meanwhile, in a bowl combine the ricotta cheese, spinach, Parmesan cheese, egg, basil, and nutmeg. Mix well.

3 Drain the shells. Spoon equal amounts of filling into each shell and place them filling-side up in the prepared baking pan. Spoon the remaining marinara sauce on top.

4 Cover with foil and bake for about 35–40 minutes. Uncover and sprinkle with the mozzarella cheese. Bake for 5–10 minutes until cheese is melted.

EXCHANGES/ CHOICES		
1 1/2 Starch 1 Med-Fat Meat	Calories **180** Calories from Fat **35** Total Fat **4.0 g** Saturated Fat **1.7 g** Trans Fat **0.0 g** Cholesterol **50 mg**	Sodium **395 mg** Total Carbohydrate **23 g** Dietary Fiber **2 g** Sugars **8 g** Protein **14 g**

A Pasta Primer

Pasta di semola grano duro indicates the pasta is made from durum wheat flour; that's the best flour for pasta.

The word endings to pasta sizes indicate the size of the shape: ONI is large (rigatoni) and ETTE or ETTI indicates small (spaghetti). INI are smaller still.

Although "fresh" pasta may imply greater nutritional value, both fresh and dried are just about the same nutritionally.

It's all in the name—here's what they mean:

CAPELLI D'ANGELO
Angel hair—long, extremely thin strands

CANNELLONI
Large tubes, filled and baked

CONCHIGLIE
Shells

DITTALI
Thimbles or tubes, ditalini are very small ones used in soups

FARFALLE
Bows or butterflies

FETTUCCINI
Long flat ribbons, about 1/4-inch wide

FUSILLI
Spirals or corkscrews. They can be long or short. Another name is rotini.

Tagliatelle with Creamy Goat Cheese Sauce

12 ounces tagliatelle or other long-stranded pasta

1/2 cup part-skim ricotta cheese

4 ounces soft, mild, reduced-fat goat cheese

6 scallions, thinly sliced

kosher salt, to taste

freshly ground black pepper, to taste

1/4 cup chopped toasted walnuts

By using both ricotta and goat cheese mixed with a little pasta water, you can produce a creamy lower-fat sauce for just about any pasta. You would think that with this few ingredients, this recipe wouldn't amount to much. On the contrary, less is more; more flavor, that is!

1 Cook the pasta in lightly salted boiling water until al dente, about 10 minutes. Drain, reserving about 1/2 cup of the pasta cooking water.

2 Mix together the ricotta and goat cheeses. Add the pasta cooking water and mix until a smooth sauce forms. Toss the sauce with the cooked pasta and mix in the scallions. Season with salt and pepper. Transfer to a serving bowl or platter and top with the walnuts.

EXCHANGES/ CHOICES		
1 1/2 Starch 1 Med-Fat Meat	Calories **255** Calories from Fat **70**	Sodium **85 mg** Total Carbohydrate **35 g** Dietary Fiber **2 g** Sugars **2 g**
	Total Fat **8.0 g** Saturated Fat **2.5 g** Trans Fat **0.0 g**	Protein **11 g**
	Cholesterol **40 mg**	

GEMELLI
Narrow spirals with hollow ends

GNOCCHI
Fluted shells. Also known as cavatelli

LASAGNE
Flat, rectangular or square sheets

LINGUINE
Long, flat ribbon noodles that are thinner than fettuccine

LUMACHE
Snail-shaped pasta

MACARONI
Smooth, thick tubes. They can be long or short, straight or curved. Cavatappi are ridged spiral macaroni.

ORECCHIETTE
Small ear-shaped pasta

PAPPARADELLE
Flat noodles that are 3/4-inch wide

PENNE
Short, straight tubes, ridged or smooth

RIGATONI
Short, ridged tubes fatter than penne

SPAGHETTI
The most familiar of the pastas, long string-like strands

TAGLIATELLE
Long flat ribbons very similar to fettuccine

VERMICELLI
A thinner and finer version of spaghetti

Classic Cheesecake, p. 154

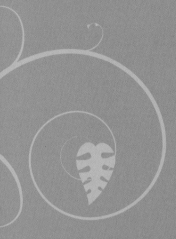

CHAPTER 8
Desserts

Almond Biscotti | 144

Ambrosia | 145

Apple Pandowdy | 147

Apple Blueberry Almond Crisp | 148

Baked Apples with Figs | 149

Chunky Applesauce | 150

Banana Chocolate Chip Muffins | 151

Chocolate Cherry Pudding | 152

Classic Cheesecake | 154

Double Chocolate Brownies | 156

Fudge Pudding Cake | 158

Lemon Scones | 159

Pear-Raisin Streusel Crunch Pie | 160

Old Fashioned Peanut Butter Cookies | 162

Plum Clafouti | 163

Raspberry Ice Cream Floats | 164

Tapioca Rice and Rhubarb Pudding | 165

Triple Gingerbread Squares | 167

Vanilla Angel Cake | 168

Vanilla Custard with Blueberry Sauce | 169

Almond Biscotti

2 cups all-purpose flour

1/3 cup sugar

3 tablespoons stevia

1 1/2 teaspoons baking powder

1 teaspoon cinnamon

6 ounces whole blanched almonds

3 large eggs

2 teaspoons vanilla extract

The first time I learned how to make proper biscotti was on a farm in Tuscany. My instructor told me true biscotti does not use any fat except for the fat in the eggs and nuts. So no butter or oils are necessary at all. Biscotti should be hard enough make them go crunch in your mouth, but no so hard that you break a tooth! Dip this in a favorite cup of coffee for a special treat.

1 Set a rack in the middle of the oven and preheat to 350°F.

2 In a bowl, combine the flour, sugar, stevia, baking powder, and cinnamon and stir well to mix. Stir in the almonds.

3 In another bowl, whisk the eggs and the vanilla extract. Add to the dry ingredients and stir until stiff dough is formed.

4 Scrape the dough onto a lightly floured surface and divide in half. Roll each half into a cylinder, just a bit shorter than the baking sheet. Place the dough onto the baking sheet covered with parchment paper. Press down gently with the palm of your hand to flatten the logs.

5 Bake for 25 to 30 minutes until they feel firm to the touch. Place on a rack and let cool for 10 minutes.

6 Once the logs have cooled, using a serrated knife, slice each log into diagonally cut pieces about 1/3-inch thick. Arrange the cookies on prepared pans, cut side down. Bake the cookies for about 15 minutes until well toasted. Cool completely.

EXCHANGES/ CHOICES		
1/2 Carbohydrate 1/2 Fat	Calories **70**	Sodium **20 mg**
	Calories from Fat **25**	Total Carbohydrate **8 g**
	Total Fat **3.0 g**	Dietary Fiber **1 g**
	Saturated Fat **0.4 g**	Sugars **2 g**
	Trans Fat **0.0 g**	Protein **2 g**
	Cholesterol **20 mg**	

Ambrosia

1 tablespoon honey

2 teaspoons fresh lime juice

3 peeled and sectioned clementine oranges

1/2 cup diced fresh apples

1/4 cup flaked coconut

2 tablespoons dried cranberries

Ambrosia is usually riddled with mini marshmallows and/or some kind of cream. This is a clean, streamlined version of Ambrosia that is a lot healthier. We used to make ambrosia all the time for guests of our family. I've slimmed down the recipe, but it's still got the same great flavor combinations of the original.

1   Mix together the honey and lime juice in the bottom of a serving bowl. Add in the oranges, apples, coconut, and cranberries and mix well.

EXCHANGES/ CHOICES		
1 Carbohydrate	Calories **85**	Sodium **15 mg**
	Calories from Fat **15**	Total Carbohydrate **19 g**
	Total Fat **1.5 g**	Dietary Fiber **2 g**
	Saturated Fat **1.2 g**	Sugars **15 g**
	Trans Fat **0.0 g**	Protein **1 g**
	Cholesterol **0 mg**	

A Little Chocolate Goes a Long Way

A small amount of melted chocolate topping a dessert is a lovely way to end a meal. Plan on no more than 1/2 ounce of chocolate per person and buy the best chocolate you can afford. Place chopped chocolate in a microwave-safe bowl, microwave at 30-second intervals, stirring between each interval until melted.

• Add melted chocolate to part-skim ricotta cheese with a small amount of stevia, Splenda, or another low-calorie sweetener, or just sugar. Mix well and use a spoonful as a topping on cakes and pies.

• Dip a marshmallow in melted chocolate and roll in chopped nuts. One marsh-mallow is equal to one serving.

• Dip half a dried apricot or half a fresh banana in melted chocolate. Set the fruit on a waxed paper lined tray. Set in the refrigerator and let dry until the chocolate is hard.

Apple Pandowdy, p. 147

Apple Pandowdy

APPLES

3 pounds firm baking apples

2 tablespoons fresh lemon juice

1/3 cup packed brown sugar

1/4 cup stevia

1/4 cup all-purpose flour

1 teaspoon ground cinnamon

BISCUITS

1 1/4 cups flour

1 1/3 tablespoons sugar

1 tablespoon stevia

1 teaspoon baking powder

1/4 teaspoon salt

1 egg

1 tablespoon melted butter

1 teaspoon vanilla extract

1/3 cup fat-free milk

This dessert is perfect for the fall. I love apple desserts because they are a great way to get to know seasonal apple varieties. I really enjoy going to farmers' markets and asking vendors which apples they like to use in different desserts. Use a mix of different types of apples in apple desserts so that you can get different flavor notes and different textures. For this fragrant pandowdy, I used half Golden Delicious and half Honey Crisps. Granny Smith, Pink Lady, Jonathan, or Northern Spy varieties also work well here.

1 Preheat the oven to 400°F. Peel and core apples, and slice into 1/4-inch thick slices. In a large bowl, combine apple slices, lemon juice, brown sugar, 1/4 cup stevia, 1/4 cup flour, and cinnamon. Toss well. Transfer to a 2 1/2-quart baking pan.

2 In a medium bowl, combine 1 1/4 cups flour with the sugar, stevia, baking powder, and salt. Make a well in the center and add the egg, butter, vanilla, and milk. Quickly incorporate the liquid ingredients into the dry, just until blended.

3 Spoon the dough into free-form biscuits over the apples. Bake for 35–40 minutes until the topping is golden and the fruit is bubbly.

EXCHANGES/CHOICES	Calories **130**	Sodium **85 mg**
	Calories from Fat **15**	Total Carbohydrate **28 g**
2 Carbohydrate	Total Fat **1.5 g**	Dietary Fiber **2 g**
	Saturated Fat **0.7 g**	Sugars **15 g**
	Trans Fat **0.0 g**	Protein **2 g**
	Cholesterol **15 mg**	

SERVES 8 SERVING SIZE 1/8 recipe PREPARATION TIME 25 minutes COOK TIME 15 minutes

Apple Blueberry Almond Crisp

TOPPING

1 tablespoon all-purpose flour

1 2/3 tablespoons unsalted butter, cold

2 tablespoons brown sugar

1/4 cup oatmeal

1 tablespoon toasted sliced almonds

1 tablespoon homemade breadcrumbs (use whole-wheat or multigrain bread)

FILLING

2 Granny Smith apples, peeled, cored, and sliced thin

1/2 cup blueberries (fresh or use frozen wild blueberries)

2 tablespoons unsweetened applesauce

1/2 teaspoon cinnamon

1/2 teaspoon vanilla

1 teaspoon lemon zest

Adding blueberries to the traditional apple crisp adds a bit more color and the berry juice makes the crisp very moist. By using ramekins, you have a completely portion-controlled satisfying serving. I like Granny Smith apples best, but feel free to use any type of apple except Red Delicious; they do not cook up well.

1 Preheat oven to 400°F. Prepare eight 2-inch ramekins with butter-flavored nonstick spray.

2 Mix flour, butter, and brown sugar in a food processor and pulse 10–15 times to make a crumbly mix. Put in a small bowl and store in freezer until ready to use.

3 Mix oatmeal, toasted almonds, and homemade breadcrumbs in a food processor and pulse 10 times, or until coarse. Add to the brown sugar mix and store in the freezer until ready to use.

4 In a small saucepan, add apples, blueberries, applesauce, cinnamon, vanilla, and zest of lemon. Cook over medium heat until apples begin to soften and the blueberries burst, about 5–7 minutes.

5 Add filling to ramekins and add topping. Bake on the center rack for 15 minutes.

EXCHANGES/CHOICES

1 Carbohydrate
1/2 Fat

Calories **80**
 Calories from Fat **25**
Total Fat **3.0 g**
 Saturated Fat **1.8 g**
 Trans Fat **0.0 g**
Cholesterol **5 mg**

Sodium **0 mg**
Total Carbohydrate **14 g**
 Dietary Fiber **1 g**
 Sugars **9 g**
Protein **1 g**

Baked Apples with Figs

1 tablespoon agave nectar

1 tablespoon brown sugar

1 teaspoon ground cinnamon

1 teaspoon vanilla

2 medium apples, peeled and chopped into 1/2-inch pieces

6 fresh figs, stemmed and chopped into 1/2-inch pieces

1/4 cup fat-free granola

Adding figs to a classic Baked Apple recipe jazzes it up. Apples take on a creamy texture that is so soothing. Low-fat granola gives it much-needed crunch. Fiddle around with the quantity of cinnamon you want—the aroma in your kitchen will be heavenly!

1 Preheat the oven to 350°F. Combine the agave nectar, brown sugar, cinnamon, and vanilla in a bowl and mix well. Add in the apples and figs and toss to coat.

2 Add the mixture to an 8 × 8-inch baking pan and sprinkle with the granola. Cover with foil and bake for 25 minutes until the apples are tender.

3 Remove the cover and bake for 5 minutes until the top is browned.

EXCHANGES/ CHOICES

1 1/2 Carbohydrate

Calories **90**
 Calories from Fat **0**
Total Fat **0.0 g**
 Saturated Fat **0.1 g**
 Trans Fat **0.0 g**
Cholesterol **0 mg**

Sodium **15 mg**
Total Carbohydrate **23 g**
 Dietary Fiber **3 g**
 Sugars **13 g**
Protein **1 g**

Baking with Bananas

Either bananas are too green or too past their prime. Here's how to get them ready for luscious baking.

• Store greenish bananas with some ripe apples. The apples give off ethylene gas, which speeds up ripening. Add the banana bunch with 2 apples in a brown paper bag, close the bag, and let ripen overnight on the kitchen counter.

• If you need ripe bananas even faster, add them unpeeled to a baking sheet. Bake at 400°F until the skin blackens. Peel, let cool, and use in your recipe.

• Don't store already ripe bananas in a fruit arrangement that contains apples. They will over ripen quickly.

Chunky Applesauce

4 large (8 ounces each) baking apples, peeled and diced

3 tablespoons sugar

2 tablespoons fresh lemon juice

1/2 teaspoon ground cinnamon

1/4 teaspoon ground ginger

Never made your own applesauce before? Try this recipe and you'll give up bottled applesauce forever. Use Jonathan or Rome apples for best results. And keep it a little chunky; it's a palate stimulator!

1   Combine all ingredients n a medium saucepan. Cover and cook over low heat, stirring often for about 10–15 minutes.

2   Lightly mash with a potato masher or immersion blender. Chill in the refrigerator or serve warm.

EXCHANGES/ CHOICES

1 1/2 Carbohydrate

Calories **85**
   Calories from Fat **0**
Total Fat **0.0 g**
   Saturated Fat **0.0 g**
   Trans Fat **0.0 g**
Cholesterol **0 mg**

Sodium **0 mg**
Total Carbohydrate **22 g**
   Dietary Fiber **2 g**
   Sugars **18 g**
Protein **0 g**

A little flavoring goes a long way...

A little flavoring gives zest and variety to your desserts. Try these variations in puddings, cakes, breads, and cookies.

ALCOHOL While people with diabetes should watch their alcohol intake, just a spoonful of rum, brandy, or sherry will enhance the flavor of fruit desserts or add a teaspoon to quick breads for a burst of flavor.

CHOCOLATE While chocolate is high in calories, sugar, and fat, it also provides antioxidants that can support good health. Just a tad of good quality chocolate is needed to add richness to baking. Look for chocolate that has a high percent of cocoa (60% or more), as these contain less fat and sugar. Using a Dutch processed cocoa in baking provides a much richer flavor than conventional cocoas and will give baked goods a rich dark color.

HERBS AND SPICES Try adding dried basil, thyme, or marjoram to scones and muffins. Make sure the dried herbs are still potent, in your pantry for less than 1 year. Add a pinch of ground chili to a recipe with chocolate for a slight savory flavor.

SALT The amount of salt you will add to a baked good is so small, but makes such a difference. Salt actually brings out the sweet flavors in baked goods, so this improves the overall flavor.

And home-baked desserts with salt added contain far less than commercially prepared ones.

VANILLA Good quality vanilla makes all the difference. Make sure that you buy pure real vanilla, not imitation vanilla. The best vanilla comes from Madagascar or Mexico. For some of the best vanilla I've ever had, go online and purchase from www.penzeys.com.

Banana Chocolate Chip Muffins

4 ripe medium bananas

2 eggs

1/2 cup brown sugar

1/3 cup plain nonfat yogurt

1/2 cup 1% milk

1/4 cup canola oil

1 3/4 cups all-purpose flour

2 teaspoons baking powder

3/4 teaspoon baking soda

1 teaspoon ground cinnamon

1/4 teaspoon salt

1/4 cup mini chocolate chips

A good chef friend of mine taught me that the secret to great banana flavor in baked goods is to actually roast whole bananas in their skin until the skin blackens. This technique gives the entire muffin a roasted caramel flavor.

1 Preheat the oven to 350°F. Coat 16 muffin cups with cooking spray.*

2 Add the unpeeled, whole bananas to a large baking sheet. Roast the bananas for about 20 minutes until the skins turn black. Remove the bananas from the oven and allow to cool enough to handle. Peel the bananas, discard the skins, and remove any stringiness from the bananas. Mash the bananas in a bowl. Set aside.

3 In a medium bowl, whisk together the eggs, sugar, yogurt, milk, and oil until smooth.

4 In a large bowl, mix together the flour, baking powder, baking soda, cinnamon, and salt.

5 Make a well in the center of the flour mixture and add the egg sugar mixture. Mix well, but do not overbeat. Fold in the bananas and chocolate chips and mix for 1 minute.

6 Fill each prepared muffin cup two-thirds full with the banana muffin batter. Bake the muffins for about 20–25 minutes or until a tester inserted in the center of a muffin comes out clean.

7 Remove the muffins from the oven and let cool for 5 minutes in the pan. Turn out the muffins to a cooling rack and cool completely. Store in a covered container.

*Add water to any muffin cups (half full) that will not be filled with batter to prevent the unused cups from burning.

EXCHANGES/ CHOICES	Calories **160**	Sodium **160 mg**
	Calories from Fat **45**	Total Carbohydrate **27 g**
2 Carbohydrate 1/2 Fat	Total Fat **5.0 g**	Dietary Fiber **1 g**
	Saturated Fat **1.0 g**	Sugars **13 g**
	Trans Fat **0.0 g**	Protein **3 g**
	Cholesterol **25 mg**	

Chocolate Cherry Pudding

3 tablespoons flour

3 tablespoons cornstarch

1/4 cup sugar

1/4 cup stevia

pinch salt

3 cups 1% milk

2 ounces semi-sweet
chocolate, finely
chopped

1 large egg

2 teaspoons vanilla

2 cups fresh or frozen
(thawed) pitted cherries,
halved

Chocolate and cherries—what a combo! It was my husband who actually got me hooked on the sweet dark cherries and chocolate taste. I would definitely serve this for company.

1 In a medium saucepan, whisk together the flour, cornstarch, sugar, stevia, and salt. Whisk in the milk until well incorporated, making sure to scrape the corners of the saucepan. Bring to a gentle simmer over medium heat, stirring frequently. Add in 1 ounce of chocolate. Simmer for 2 minutes until the pudding has thickened slightly.

2 In a small bowl, lightly beat the egg, gradually beat 3/4 cup of the hot pudding into the egg, then whisk the egg mixture back into the pan and cook for 1 minute. Remove from the heat and stir in the vanilla. Pour the pudding into a bowl and cover with plastic wrap directly on the surface of the pudding. Cool to room temperature and then refrigerate for 30 minutes. Stir in all except 4 teaspoons of the remaining chocolate. Mix in the cherries.

3 Add the pudding to 8 individual dessert cups. Sprinkle each cup with 1/2 teaspoon of chopped chocolate.

EXCHANGES/
CHOICES

1 Carbohydrate
1/2 Fat

Calories **105**
  Calories from Fat **25**

Total Fat **3.0 g**
  Saturated Fat **1.4 g**
  Trans Fat **0.0 g**

Cholesterol **20 mg**

Sodium **35 mg**

Total Carbohydrate **18 g**
  Dietary Fiber **1 g**
  Sugars **13 g**

Protein **3 g**

Chocolate Cherry Pudding, p. 152

Classic Cheesecake

CRUST

1 cup graham cracker crumbs (approximately 8–9 graham crackers)

2 tablespoons butter, melted

1/2 tablespoon stevia

1 tablespoon sugar

1 teaspoon ground cinnamon

FILLING

1 pound low-fat (1%) cottage cheese, drained for 10 hours*

1 pound Greek plain nonfat yogurt

1 pound fat-free cream cheese

1/4 cup plus 2 tablespoons stevia

1/4 cup plus 2 tablespoons sugar

1 tablespoon vanilla extract

1/4 teaspoon salt

3 large eggs

TOPPING

1 cup sliced strawberries

I would not let this book be published if I did not come up with a cheesecake recipe. And being a native New Yorker, cheesecake is abasic staple comfort food. It's creamy, silky, everything you have come to expect from cheesecake except putting on a few pounds after indulging.

1 Preheat the oven to 325°F. Position an oven rack to the middle of the oven.

2 Combine the graham cracker crumbs, melted butter, 1/2 tablespoon stevia, 1 tablespoon sugar, and cinnamon. Press the crumb mixture evenly into the bottom of a 9-inch springform pan. Bake the crust for 8 minutes. Remove from the oven and set on a rack to cool.

3 Increase the oven temperature to 500°F. Add the cottage cheese to a food processor and process until very smooth. Add the yogurt and cream cheese and process for another 1–2 minutes until smooth. Add in the stevia, sugar, vanilla, and salt and process until smooth. With the processor running, add the eggs, one at a time and process until incorporated.

4 Add the batter to the prepared crust. Bake the cheesecake for about 8 minutes. Lower the temperature to 200°F and bake until the cheesecake is set, about 1 hour.

EXCHANGES/ CHOICES		
1 Carbohydrate 1 Lean Meat 1/2 Fat	Calories **135**	Sodium **400 mg**
	Calories from Fat 25	Total Carbohydrate **14 g**
	Total Fat **3.0 g**	Dietary Fiber **0 g**
	Saturated Fat **1.5 g**	Sugars **10 g**
	Trans Fat **0.0 g**	Protein **11 g**
	Cholesterol **50 mg**	

*Instead of draining the cottage cheese for 10 hours, you can absorb the extra moisture with paper towels. Place two layers of paper towels on a plate, place the cottage cheese on top, and place another two layers of paper towel on top of the cottage cheese. Press down on the cottage cheese so the paper towels absorb any extra liquid it may have. Discard the top layers of paper towel and use a large spoon to transfer the cottage cheese to the food processor. Discard the bottom layers of paper towel.

5 Transfer the cake to a wire rack. Run a paring knife around the edge of the cake to loosen it. Cool completely at room temperature, about 2–3 hours. Cover with plastic wrap and refrigerate for 3 hours or overnight.

6 Remove the sides of the pan and let the cheesecake come to room temperature for about 30 minutes. Decorate the top with sliced strawberries. Slice and serve.

Fruit Purée Substitutes

As you fiddle with your own dessert recipes, think about how you can reduce the fat and sugar. By using fruit purées you can add moisture, delicious flavor, and natural sweetness. Fruit purées are best in quick breads.

- A simple formula is to replace half the fat and half the sugar with the same weight of fruit purée. Experiment with the ratio until you find the texture that you like.

- For darker, richer cakes like chocolate cake, make a dried fruit purée and substitute it for the same weight of fat and sugar in a recipe: Add about 4 ounces of dried prunes, apricots, or apples and put them in a pan with water to cover. Cover and simmer on low heat until very soft. Purée in a blender or food processor.

- For lighter colored cakes, like banana or carrot, make an apple purée and substitute it for the same weight of fat and sugar in a recipe. Peel, core, and thinly slice baking apples such as Jonathan or McIntosh and use about 2 tablespoons of water per apple to cover. Cover and simmer on very low heat for 30 minutes, until tender. Mash or purée in food processor.

Double Chocolate Brownies

2/3 cup all-purpose flour

1/3 cup Dutch process cocoa (such as Droste)

1 teaspoon baking powder

1/4 teaspoon salt

1/4 cup bittersweet chocolate chips (such as Ghirardelli)

1 tablespoon butter

1/4 cup granulated sugar

1/4 cup brown sugar

3 tablespoons reduced-fat sour cream

1 tablespoon unsweetened applesauce

1 tablespoon fat-free chocolate syrup

1 egg

1 egg white

2 teaspoons pure vanilla extract

This brownie is moist and cakey. Using too much applesauce can cause baked products to become slick and gummy. But this brownie has a perfect balance of a little fat from pure butter, plus low-fat sour cream, fat-free chocolate syrup, and just 1 tablespoon of applesauce to keep the brownies fudgy and addicting.

1 Preheat the oven to 325°F. Coat an 8 × 8-inch baking pan with cooking spray. Set aside.

2 In a medium bowl, mix together the flour, cocoa powder, baking powder, and salt. Set aside.

3 In a microwave-safe container, add the chocolate chips and butter. Microwave for 1 minute. Remove from the microwave carefully and stir the mixture until it is smooth. Add the melted chocolate mixture to a large bowl. Let cool for 5 minutes. If a microwave is not available, heat a small saucepan with 1/4 cup water, bring to a simmer. Put a mixing bowl on top and add the chocolate chips and butter. Stir mixture until melted, about 5 minutes. Add the melted chocolate to a large bowl, let cool for 5 minutes.

4 Add the sugars, sour cream, applesauce, chocolate syrup, egg, egg white, and vanilla to the melted chocolate mixture and stir until well combined. Slowly add the flour in thirds to the chocolate mixture. Do not overbeat; mix until just combined.

EXCHANGES/ CHOICES		
1 Carbohydrate	Calories **65**	Sodium **60 mg**
	Calories from Fat **20**	Total Carbohydrate **11 g**
	Total Fat **2.0 g**	Dietary Fiber **1 g**
	Saturated Fat **1.2 g**	Sugars **7 g**
	Trans Fat **0.0 g**	Protein **1 g**
	Cholesterol **15 mg**	

5   Pour the mixture into the prepared pan. Position the oven rack to the lower third of the oven. Bake the brownies for 15 minutes. Insert a tester. The brownies should look slightly under-baked and the top should look fudgy.

6   Remove the pan from the oven and place on a wire rack. Let the brownies cool for 2 hours in the pan. The brownies will firm up a bit. Cut into 20 squares.

OPTIONAL GLAZE

1/4 cup half-and-half

1 cup bittersweet chocolate chips

1   In a small saucepan, add the half-and-half and chocolate chips and melt until smooth.

2   Spread the glaze over the brownies. Let the glaze set for 30 minutes. Cut the brownies into 20 squares. (Not included in nutrition analysis.)

Fudge Pudding Cake

CAKE LAYER

3/4 cup all-purpose flour

1/2 cup stevia

1/4 cup sugar

1/4 teaspoon salt

1/2 cup fat-free milk

2 teaspoons butter

4 teaspoons light butter
(such as Land O' Lakes)

1 square unsweetened
chocolate, melted

1 1/2 teaspoons baking
powder

1 teaspoon vanilla extract

PUDDING LAYER

1/2 cup brown sugar

1/4 cup stevia

3 tablespoons Dutch
process cocoa

pinch salt

1 1/2 cups boiling water

Chocolate cake that forms its own rich, fudgy sauce is a true comfort food dessert. When I was a kid, we made this all the time on rainy days. My updated version is slimmed down, but retains all the concentrated chocolate flavor you could hope for.

1   Preheat the oven to 350°F. For the cake layer, in a large bowl, combine the flour, stevia, sugar, salt, milk, butter, chocolate, baking powder, and vanilla extract. Mix at low speed with an electric mixer until just mixed. Increase the speed to medium and beat about 4 minutes, scraping the bowl occasionally. Don't worry; the batter will look slightly curdled.

2   Pour the batter into an 8 × 8-inch baking dish.

3   To prepare the pudding layer, combine the brown sugar, stevia, cocoa, and salt and sprinkle over the cake layer. Pour boiling water over all and do not stir. Bake for 35–40 minutes. Cool slightly, serve warm.

EXCHANGES/ CHOICES	Calories **140**	Sodium **145 mg**
	Calories from Fat **30**	Total Carbohydrate **27 g**
2 Carbohydrate	Total Fat **3.5 g**	Dietary Fiber **1 g**
	Saturated Fat **2.0 g**	Sugars **17 g**
	Trans Fat **0.0 g**	Protein **2 g**
	Cholesterol **5 mg**	

Lemon Scones

2 cups all-purpose flour

1/4 cup stevia

2 teaspoons baking powder

1/2 teaspoon baking soda

1/4 teaspoon salt

1/2 cup buttery spread (such as Promise Activ)

1 cup dried currants or coarsely chopped dried cranberries

2 teaspoons grated lemon zest

1/2–3/4 cup low-fat buttermilk

Rich and crumbly, these taste exactly like what you would get from a corner bakery shop. The important difference is that the fat is kept to a minimum, but you get the look, taste, and texture of the high-fat versions. Make these either with currants or, for an eye-popping look, use dried cranberries instead.

1   Preheat the oven to 400°F. Coat a large baking sheet with cooking spray.

2   In a bowl, combine the flour, stevia, baking powder, baking soda, and salt. Cut in the buttery spread until the mixture resembles coarse crumbs. Add in the currants and lemon zest.

3   Add in enough buttermilk to form a soft dough. Turn the dough out on a floured surface. Knead lightly 4–5 times.

4   Roll the dough out to a 1/2-inch thickness. Cut into 8 triangular pieces. Place the scones on the baking sheet and bake for 10–12 minutes until lightly browned.

EXCHANGES/ CHOICES		
2 1/2 Carbohydrate	Calories **215**	Sodium **305 mg**
1 Fat	Calories from Fat **40**	Total Carbohydrate **41 g**
	Total Fat **4.5 g**	Dietary Fiber **2 g**
	Saturated Fat **0.6 g**	Sugars **15 g**
	Trans Fat **0.0 g**	Protein **5 g**
	Cholesterol **0 mg**	

Pear-Raisin Streusel Crunch Pie

PIE CRUST

1 1/4 cups all-purpose flour

1 teaspoon stevia

1/4 teaspoon salt

3 tablespoons margarine (such as Promise Buttery Spread) or butter, chilled and cut into pieces

1 tablespoon canola oil

1 teaspoon cider vinegar

4 tablespoons ice water

1 egg white, lightly beaten

FILLING

4 medium-sized ripe Bartlett pears, cored and thinly sliced

1/2 cup raisins

1 teaspoon stevia

1 teaspoon vanilla

1 tablespoon flour

1/2 teaspoon ground cinnamon

This simple raisin and pear pie is perfect when there is an abundance of pears at your farmer's market or grocer. The low-fat crust is easy to prepare and very flaky and you'll love the granola-like topping. This is a great pie for informal get-togethers as well as any holiday affair.

1 For pie crust: add the flour, stevia, and salt to the bowl of a food processor. Mix well to combine. Add the butter or margarine and pulse mixer until coarse crumbs form. Combine the oil, vinegar, and water and drizzle over the dry ingredients. Pulse mixer until crumbs are moistened.

2 Pour dough out onto a piece of plastic wrap (mixture will be crumbly). Gently press crumbs into a 1/2-inch-thick circle and wrap tightly in plastic wrap. Refrigerate for 30 minutes.

3 Place dough on a lightly floured surface and roll out into a circle that is about 9 inches in diameter. Gently place the dough in an 8-inch pie plate. Press into the bottom of the pan and form a decorative border by tucking the extra dough under, around the edge, and then crimping with your fingers. (If dough tears, press back together using fingertips.)

4 Chill pie shell in refrigerator for at least 30 minutes before filling.

5 For filling: place all filling ingredients in a large bowl and toss well to coat. Set aside.

EXCHANGES/ CHOICES		
3 Carbohydrate 1 1/2 Fat	Calories **280** Calories from Fat **70** Total Fat **8.0 g** Saturated Fat **0.9 g** Trans Fat **0.0 g** Cholesterol **0 mg**	Sodium **175 mg** Total Carbohydrate **49 g** Dietary Fiber **5 g** Sugars **17 g** Protein **5 g**

STREUSEL TOPPING

1 cup oatmeal

1/4 cup flour

2 tablespoons stevia

1 tablespoon brown sugar

1 teaspoon cinnamon

1/8 teaspoon salt

2 tablespoon margarine (such as Promise Buttery Spread) or butter, chilled and cut into pieces

1/4 cup apple cider

6 For streusel topping: combine the oatmeal, flour, stevia, brown sugar, cinnamon, and salt in a large bowl and stir well with a whisk. Using a pastry blender or two knives, cut in the margarine or butter until coarse crumbs form. Add the apple cider and mix until it is like granola.

7 Preheat oven to 400°F. Prick pie shell, brush the bottom of the crust with the beaten egg white all over with a fork so steam can escape. Arrange fruit filling in the crust and sprinkle evenly with streusel topping. Bake for 20 minutes and reduce oven temperature to 350°F. Bake at reduced heat for an additional 30 to 35 minutes, until the crust is golden and the fruit is tender when tested with a knife. Cool pie slightly and serve at room temperature.

A Tender Crust Makes the Best Pie

- Use very cold water to make pastry dough; ice water is even better. Pour water into a glass of ice cubes and let it stand for a minute or so. Measure the water needed by pouring it out from the glass.

- Chill the rolling pin and board.
- Chill the pastry at least 30 minutes prior to rolling it out.
- Use a marble slab for rolling the dough out so it stays cool.

- Handle the dough as little as possible.
- Use dark metal pans for pie crusts. Since they absorb heat, the crusts will brown faster and more evenly.

Old Fashioned Peanut Butter Cookies

2/3 cup packed brown sugar

1/4 cup stevia

3 tablespoons butter

2 1/2 tablespoons non-hydrogenated buttery spread (such as Activ or Smart Balance)

1/4 cup plus 2 tablespoons crunchy unsalted peanut butter

2 teaspoons vanilla

1 egg

3 tablespoons water

1 3/4 cup all-purpose flour

3/4 teaspoon baking soda

1/2 teaspoon salt

These peanut butter cookies are cake-like and have a wonderful peanut butter aroma and beautiful golden brown color. Bet you can't eat just one!

1   Preheat the oven to 350°F. Line 2 baking sheets with parchment paper.

2   In a medium bowl, cream together the brown sugar, stevia, butter, buttery spread, and peanut butter until smooth. Add the vanilla, egg, and water. Beat until combined.

3   In another bowl, combine the flour, baking soda, and salt. Stir the flour mixture into the peanut butter mixture.

4   Shape the batter into 1-inch balls and place them on the prepared baking sheets, leaving a 2-inch space between each cookie. Using a fork that has been dipped in water, flatten the cookies, making a cross-hatched pattern.

5   Bake the cookies for 8–10 minutes until the cookies are just set. Remove the cookies from the oven. Cool on the baking sheets for 2 minutes. Remove from the cookie sheets and let cool completely on wire racks.

EXCHANGES/ CHOICES		
1/2 Carbohydrate 1/2 Fat	Calories **70** Calories from Fat **25**	Sodium **75 mg** Total Carbohydrate **9 g**
	Total Fat **3.0 g** Saturated Fat **0.9 g** Trans Fat **0.0 g**	Dietary Fiber **0 g** Sugars **4 g**
	Cholesterol **10 mg**	Protein **1 g**

Plum Clafouti

1 pound (about 5–6) fresh black plums, pitted

1/4 cup sugar, divided

1/2 cup fresh raspberries

2 tablespoons flour

3/4 cup fat-free milk

2 tablespoons stevia

2 large eggs

pinch salt

1/2 cup blanched slivered almonds

Although not an easy word to pronounce, clafouti is one of my all-time favorite comfort desserts. It's like a giant puffed pancake that contains delicious fruit. In this Plum Clafouti, beautiful ripe plums and raspberries are tucked in a light crisp batter.

1   Preheat the oven to 375°F. Slice the plums into 1/2-inch slices and add to a bowl. Toss in half the sugar and coat well. Arrange the plums in a 9-inch pie pan in concentric circles; they should make 2 layers. Scatter the raspberries over the plums.

2   In a food processor, combine the flour, milk, remaining sugar, stevia, eggs, and salt and process for 1 minute, until smooth. Pour the batter over the fruit. Scatter the almonds on top.

3   Bake for 30–35 minutes until the top is puffed and golden. Serve warm.

EXCHANGES/ CHOICES		
1 Carbohydrate 1 Fat	Calories **135** Calories from Fat **55** Total Fat **6.0 g** Saturated Fat **0.8 g** Trans Fat **0.0 g** Cholesterol **55 mg**	Sodium **30 mg** Total Carbohydrate **18 g** Dietary Fiber **2 g** Sugars **14 g** Protein **5 g**

Raspberry Ice Cream Floats

4 cups fresh raspberries

1 teaspoon stevia

1 1/2 cups no-sugar-added, reduced-fat vanilla ice cream (such as Breyers Smooth and Dreamy)

3 1/2 cups no-sodium-added club soda

This ice cream float will take you back to the simple days of summer fun. Swirls of fresh raspberries intermingle with cool vanilla ice cream all topped off with fizzy club soda. It's a malt shop favorite.

1   Press the raspberries through a fine sieve over a small bowl and discard the seeds. Combine the raspberry purée with the stevia.

2   Divide the raspberry mixture evenly among all four glasses.

3   For each glass: spoon 2 tablespoons of the ice cream into each glass on top of the raspberry purée. Stir in 2 tablespoons of the club soda. Add in about 1/2 cup more of the ice cream and pour in 3/4 cup of the club soda over ice cream. Repeat with the remaining three glasses. Serve immediately.

EXCHANGES/ CHOICES		
1 1/2 Carbohydrate 1/2 Fat	Calories **120**	Sodium **105 mg**
	Calories from Fat **35**	Total Carbohydrate **24 g**
	Total Fat **4.0 g**	Dietary Fiber **3 g**
	Saturated Fat **1.9 g**	Sugars **8 g**
	Trans Fat **0.0 g**	Protein **3 g**
	Cholesterol **20 mg**	

Quickie Nonfat Greek Yogurt Desserts

I like to use plain nonfat Greek yogurt as a dessert. Its texture is so thick and rich you really feel indulgent.

FIGS AND YOGURT

Simmer 10 chopped dried figs with 1 teaspoon honey, 1 teaspoon lemon zest, and 2 cups water for 25 minutes. Spoon 1 tablespoon of the figs over 1/2 cup yogurt.

GINGERSNAP YOGURT

Crush 5 fat-free gingersnap cookies. Mix with 1 tablespoon crystallized ginger and add to 2 cups plain yogurt (1/2 cup serving per person).

CHOCOLATE CHERRY YOGURT

Mix 1 cup fresh, pitted, or frozen and thawed Bing cherries with 2 cups plain yogurt. Spoon into 1/2 cup portions and top with 1 teaspoon grated dark chocolate.

Tapioca Rice and Rhubarb Pudding*

1/2 cup long-grain rice

1/2 cup small tapioca pearls

2 cups water

3/4 cup vanilla almond milk

1/3 cup stevia, divided

2 tablespoons sugar

1 teaspoon canola oil

2 cups chopped fresh rhubarb

1/2 cup fresh sliced strawberries

If you love sweet and tart together, then you'll love this Tapioca Rice and Rhubarb Pudding. In our house, tapioca was the best cheap comfort food ever.

1   In a saucepan, combine the rice, tapioca, and water and bring to a boil. Cook on high heat for 5–8 minutes. Add the vanilla almond milk and bring to another boil. Lower the heat, simmer on low for 20 minutes. Make sure the mixture does not get too thick; add more water if necessary to desired consistency. Add in half the stevia and all of the sugar, stir to mix well.

2   Meanwhile, heat the canola oil in a 2–3 quart saucepan over medium heat. Add the rhubarb. Cook until the rhubarb falls apart into a nice chunky sauce. Add the remaining stevia to the rhubarb. Fold in the strawberries.

3   For each serving, add 1/2 cup of the tapioca mixture to a dessert dish and top with 1/4 cup of the rhubarb sauce. Serve warm or chilled.

*Recipe courtesy of Debra Riedsel, RD

EXCHANGES/ CHOICES		
3 Carbohydrate	Calories **190**	Sodium **30 mg**
	Calories from Fat **15**	Total Carbohydrate **42 g**
	Total Fat **1.5 g**	Dietary Fiber **2 g**
	Saturated Fat **0.1 g**	Sugars **9 g**
	Trans Fat **0.0 g**	Protein **2 g**
	Cholesterol **0 mg**	

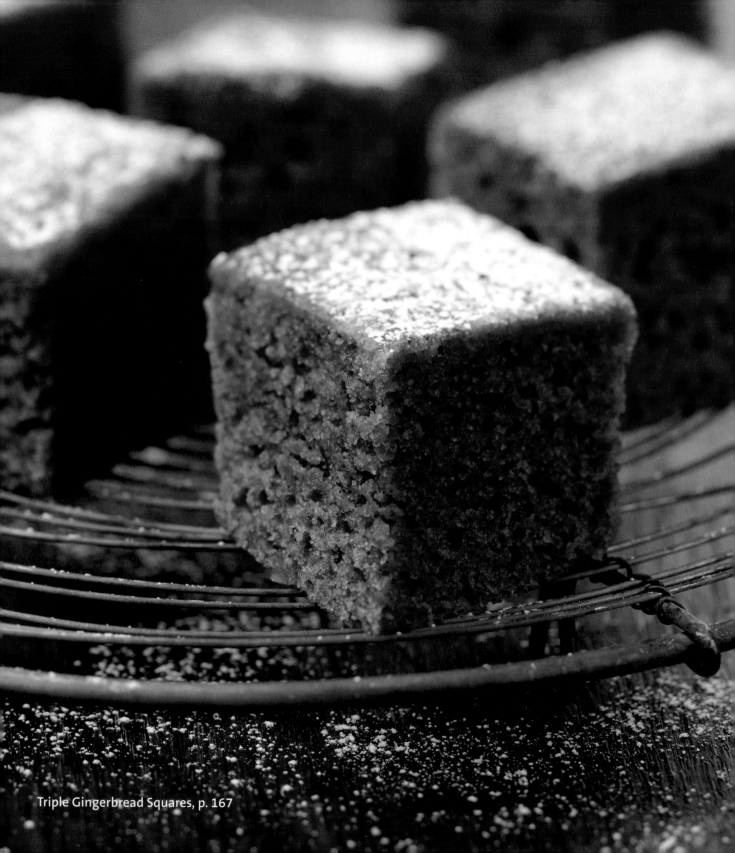

Triple Gingerbread Squares, p. 167

Triple Gingerbread Squares

1 cup all-purpose flour

1/4 cup whole-wheat pastry flour

1 tablespoon ground ginger

1/2 teaspoon ground cinnamon

1/4 teaspoon ground cloves

1/2 teaspoon baking soda

1/4 teaspoon salt

1/2 cup Splenda sugar blend

1/2 cup low-fat buttermilk

1/4 cup unsweetened applesauce

1/4 cup molasses

1/4 cup canola oil

1 egg, beaten

2 tablespoons finely minced crystallized ginger

1 teaspoon fresh-peeled finely grated ginger

1 1/2 tablespoons powdered sugar

Every year, I begin making my holiday food gifts with gingerbread. Over the years, I started using different versions and amounts of ginger. Trust me, it all works.

1 Preheat the oven to 350°F. Coat a 9-inch baking pan with cooking spray. In a large bowl, combine the flours, ground ginger, ground cinnamon, ground cloves, baking soda, and salt.

2 In another bowl, combine the Splenda with the buttermilk, applesauce, molasses, oil, egg, crystallized ginger, and fresh ginger.

3 Slowly stir in the flour mixture and mix to combine with a wire whisk.

4 Pour the batter into the prepared pan and bake for 25 minutes, or until a tester comes out clean. Cool in the pan until cool enough to cut without producing crumbs. Sprinkle with powdered sugar and cut into squares.

EXCHANGES/ CHOICES		
1 1/2 Carbohydrate	Calories **125**	Sodium **90 mg**
1/2 Fat	Calories from Fat **35**	Total Carbohydrate **20 g**
	Total Fat **4.0 g**	Dietary Fiber **1 g**
	Saturated Fat **0.4 g**	Sugars **12 g**
	Trans Fat **0.0 g**	Protein **2 g**
	Cholesterol **15 mg**	

Vanilla Angel Cake

FLOUR MIXTURE

1 1/2 cups cake flour

1/2 cup sugar

1/2 cup stevia

EGG WHITE MIXTURE

12 large egg whites, at
room temperature

1 teaspoon cream of tartar

1/2 cup stevia

1/4 teaspoon salt

1 teaspoon pure vanilla
extract

GARNISH

8 ounces strawberries, cut
into quarters

8 ounces raspberries

8 ounces blueberries

1 8-ounce container light
vanilla yogurt

When I started cutting back on fat in desserts, angel cake made frequent appearances as our after dinner treat. However, with so much sugar replacing the fat, I had another problem. But now with stevia, a natural, no-calorie sweetener, my angel food cake meets all the nutritional guidelines!

1 Coat a 10-inch tube pan with cooking spray. Preheat the oven to 350°F. Sift the flour, sugar, and stevia onto a large plate and set aside.

2 For the egg white mixture: place the egg whites and cream of tartar in a large bowl and whisk until frothy. Combine stevia and salt and add to the whipped egg whites in a slow steady stream. Add the vanilla extract, and continue whisking until the mixture forms stiff peaks.

3 Sift the flour mixture over the egg whites and fold in very gently with a large metal spoon until well blended.

4 Spoon the mixture into the prepared pan. Gently smooth the top. Bake for 35 minutes, or until golden brown and cake springs back when lightly touched in the center.

5 Invert the cake, still in pan, onto a wire rack and leave to cool completely upside down. When it is cool, slide a long knife around the side of the pan to loosen the cake and invert it onto a serving plate. The cake can be stored in an airtight container or wrapped in plastic wrap for 1–2 days.

6 Just before serving, mix together the strawberries, raspberries, and blueberries. Spoon the fruit into the hollow in the center of the cake. Serve each slice with a dollop of vanilla yogurt.

EXCHANGES/ CHOICES	Calories **140**	Sodium **100 mg**
	Calories from Fat **5**	Total Carbohydrate **29 g**
2 Carbohydrate	Total Fat **0.5 g**	Dietary Fiber **2 g**
	Saturated Fat **0.2 g**	Sugars **13 g**
	Trans Fat **0.0 g**	Protein **5 g**
	Cholesterol **0 mg**	

Vanilla Custard with Blueberry Sauce

BLUEBERRY SAUCE

4 cups fresh blueberries

1/2 cup fresh orange juice

2 tablespoons stevia

2 tablespoons sugar

1 teaspoon ground
cinnamon

rind of 1 orange

VANILLA CUSTARD

2 tablespoons arrowroot

2 cups fat-free milk,
divided

2 tablespoons stevia

2 tablespoons sugar

1 vanilla bean, split

1 egg

1 teaspoon vanilla extract

Why settle for store-bought vanilla pudding when making your own is so easy. And you can control the amount of vanilla you add in. A vanilla bean and vanilla extract are added to give a rich almost French vanilla taste to the custard. A fresh tangy blueberry sauce gives the dessert some additional nutrition and a beautiful color.

1 Combine the blueberries, orange juice, stevia, sugar, cinnamon, and the orange rind in a medium saucepan and bring to a boil over medium heat. Cover and simmer for 5 minutes.

2 In a small saucepan dissolve the arrowroot with 1/4 cup of the milk. Whisk in the stevia, sugar, and the remaining milk. Add the vanilla bean. Cook over medium heat for 5–10 minutes, until mixture comes to a boil and thickens.

3 Remove from the heat and whisk in the egg quickly. Add in the vanilla extract. Return to the heat and cook for 1 minute, stirring constantly. Strain the custard into a bowl and discard the vanilla bean. Serve the custard warm over the blueberries.

EXCHANGES/ CHOICES

2 Carbohydrate

Calories **155**
Calories from Fat **15**

Total Fat **1.5 g**
Saturated Fat **0.3 g**
Trans Fat **0.0 g**

Cholesterol **35 mg**

Sodium **45 mg**

Total Carbohydrate **32 g**
Dietary Fiber **3 g**
Sugars **24 g**

Protein **5 g**

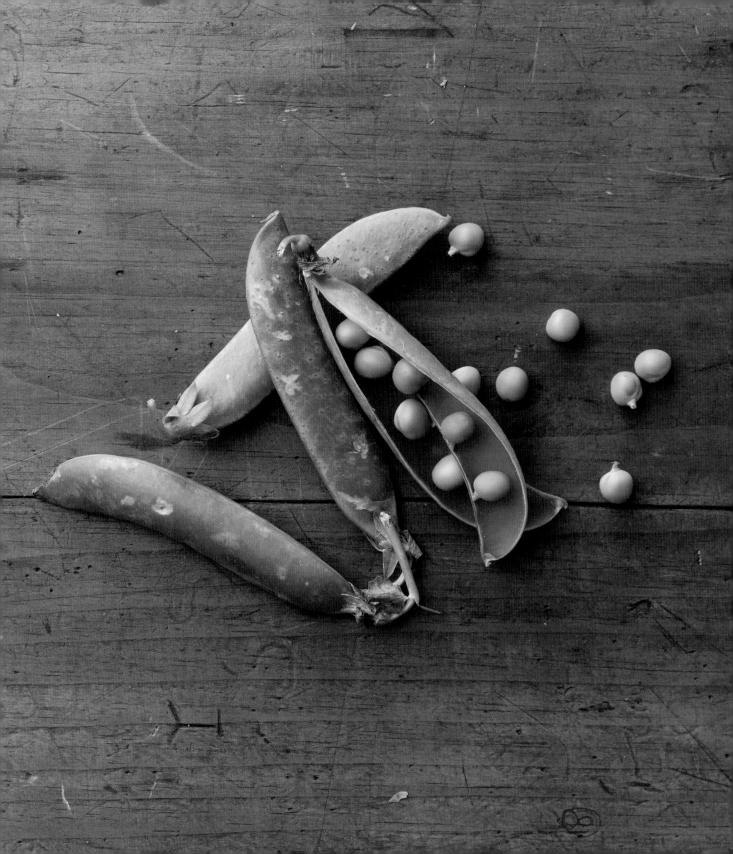

Appendix: Selecting and Storing Vegetables

Selecting and storing vegetables is easy when you take the time to search out the best produce you can find. Use these handy tips to maximize the bounty at your grocer or farmers' market.

ASPARAGUS
Choose tender, straight green stalks. Avoid spreading or woody stems. Store in plastic bags in the refrigerator crisper for 1–3 days. Best season: April to June.

GREEN BEANS
Search for smooth crisp pods. Avoid limp, wrinkled, or fat, overly mature pods. Store in plastic bags in the refrigerator crisper for 1–3 days. Available all year.

BEETS
Purchase small, unblemished beets that have small, fresh leaves and firm stems. Remove the green tops (which can be used in stir-frys or lightly sautéed in olive oil), leaving an inch or so of stem and refrigerate. Do not wash until ready to use. Available all year.

BROCCOLI
Look for dark green heads with tightly closed buds. Stalks should be tender yet firm and the leaves should be fresh and not wilted. Avoid yellow buds or rubbery stems. Store in plastic bags in the refrigerator crisper for 2–4 days. Available all year.

BRUSSELS SPROUTS
Brussels sprouts often come packed into containers, making it difficult to inspect each sprout. If possible try to find a market that sells them loose. If not, inspect the ones you can see for firm, closely curled heads with no brown spots, yellow leaves, or signs of wilt. Generally, the smaller they are, the sweeter they are. Do not wash prior to storage. Refrigerate in the original container or plastic bag and use within 3 days. Best season: August through March.

CABBAGE
Choose heads that are solid and heavy for their size. Avoid heads with splits or yellowed leaves. Store in the crisper for 3–7 days. Available all year.

CARROTS
Choose well-shaped, firm, bright orange carrots. Avoid carrots with splits or blemishes. Store in plastic bags in the crisper for 1–4 weeks. Available all year.

CAULIFLOWER

Select firm compact heads with white florets and bright green leaves. Avoid any heads with brown spots or yellowing leaves. Store in the crisper for 2–4 days. Available all year.

CELERY

Choose celery that has crisp stalks. Leaves should be light or medium green. Avoid limp or yellowed leaves. Store in the crisper for 1 week. Available all year.

GREENS

Greens for cooking, including spinach, kale, and Chinese cabbages, including bok choy, should be crisp and fresh looking, with good color, and no brown spots or yellowing leaves. Store greens in a plastic bag in the refrigerator. They keep 2–4 days, but try to use as soon after purchase as possible. Available all year.

KOHLRABI

Purchase small kohlrabi (under 2 1/2 inches in diameter). Large kohlrabi can be fibrous. Avoid ones with soft spots or a yellowish hue. Store in the refrigerator in an opened plastic bag. Since kohlrabi is a root vegetable it may also be stored in a cool dry place. Best season: mid spring to mid fall.

MUSHROOMS

Should be firm and relatively clean. Avoid bruised ones. Can be stored unwashed, loosely covered on a refrigerator shelf for 4 days. Avoid storing mushrooms in the crisper drawer as they have a tendency to become mushy. Available all year.

ONIONS

Select onions that do not appear to be ready to sprout. They should be heavy for their size. Store in a cool dry place but not in the refrigerator. Available all year.

PARSNIPS

Choose young, straight, firm roots without blemish. Avoid large roots, they tend to be woody. Store unwashed in a perforated bag in the refrigerator for 1 week. Best season: fall to winter.

BELL PEPPER

Bell peppers should be firm and well shaped with shiny flesh. Avoid limp, soft, or wrinkled peppers. Store in the crisper for 4–5 days. Available all year.

POTATOES

Look for firm, well-shaped potatoes. Avoid any that are blemished, sprouted, or cracked. Store in a cool dry place away from the sunlight. Most potatoes will keep for 2 weeks at room temperature. Available all year.

SCALLIONS

Scallions should have firm, white bulbs with crisp green tops. Avoid those with withered or yellow tops. Store in plastic bags in the refrigerator for 2–3 days. Available all year.

SHALLOTS

Choose firm, well-shaped bulbs that are heavy for their size. The papery skins should be dry and shiny. Store in a cool dry place. They will keep for several months. Available all year.

SUMMER SQUASH (ZUCCHINI AND YELLOW OR CROOKNECK SQUASH)

The youngest zucchini and yellow squash taste the best. Look for summer squash that is about 5 to 7 inches long. They should be firm and heavy for their size with tight vivid color free of brown spots or cuts. Store in a loose bag in the refrigerator. Use within 2–3 days. Best season: late spring.

TOMATOES

Tomatoes should be vine ripened and fully colored. They should feel heavy for their size. Flavor is best in tomatoes that are stored at room temperature. Avoid tomatoes from refrigerated sections of the market. Best season: late spring through early fall.

TURNIPS

Choose small, firm, slightly rounded turnips. Avoid large ones as they tend to be strong flavored and woody. Store unwashed in the refrigerator for 1 week. Available all year.

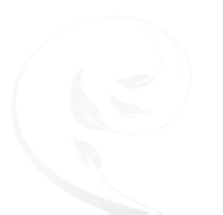

Recipe Index

NOTE: Page numbers followed by a *ph* refer to photographs.

A

Almond Biscotti, 144
Ambrosia, 145
Apple and Gorgonzola Cheese Salad, 18
Apple Blueberry Almond Crisp, 148
Apple Pandowdy, 146*ph*, 147
Asian Chicken Dumplings, 2
Asopao De Pollo- Puerto Rican Chicken and Rice Soup, 45

B

Baked Apples with Figs, 149
Baked Potato Soup, 46
Baked Turkey Meatballs, 112
Baked Ziti, 128
Banana Chocolate Chip Muffins, 151
Basil Vinegar, 40
BBQ Beef Sandwiches, 64
Black Bean Soup with a Kick, 47
Braised Cabbage and Apples, 19
Butternut Squash Stew with Chickpeas, 48

C

Caesar Salad with Chicken, 20
Caramelized Onion Chicken, 113
Cheddar Baked Potato Skins, 3
Cheddar Cheese and Broccoli Soup, 50*ph*, 51
Cheese & Fruit Bruschetta, 4
Cherry Glazed Pork Loin Chops, 114
Chicken and Noodle Salad with Peanut Dressing, 129
Chicken Cacciatore, 94
Chicken Joes, 62*ph*, 65
Chicken Paprikash, 95
Chicken Pot Pie with Phyllo, 66–67
Chicken with White Wine Garlic Sauce, 115
Chickpea Soup with Orzo, 49
Chinese Five-Spice Steak with Chinese Noodles, 96
Chocolate Cherry Pudding, 152, 153*ph*
Chocolate Cherry Yogurt, 164
Chopped Salad with Cilantro Lime Dressing, 22, 23*ph*
Chunky Applesauce, 150
Chutney Dip, 10
Clam Dip, 10
Classic Cheesecake, 142*ph*, 154–155
Classic Free-Formed Meatloaf, 68
Classic Grilled Cheese, 69
Classic Hummus, 4
Classic Mac 'n' Cheese, 70–71
Classic Ratatouille, 16*ph*, 21
Costa Rican Black Beans and Rice (Gallo Pinto), 116
Country Captain Chicken, 117
Crab Louis, 5
Creamy Crab Spread, 6
Creamy Deviled Eggs, 7
Creamy Polenta, 24
Creamy Succotash, 25
Creamy Tomato Soup, 52
Crispy Roasted Cauliflower, 26
Curry Dip, 6

D

Dill Dip, 6
Double Cheese Pizza Bites, 8
Double Chocolate Brownies, 156–157

E

Escarole and White Bean Soup, 53
Everyday Taco Salad, 72

F

Falafel, 97
Figs and Yogurt, 164
Filet Mignon with Spiced Pepper Crust, 73
5-Minute Creamy Mushroom Soup, 44
Fudge Pudding, 158

G

Garlic Vinegar, 40
Ginger Carrots with Golden Raisins and Lemon, 27
Gingersnap Yogurt, 164
Gnocchi with Tomatoes, Chickpeas, and Spinach, 98
Greek Country Salad, 28
Greek Lamb Chops, 34*ph*, 99
Grilled Lamb Burgers, 74
Grilled Pork and Cheese Quesadillas, 100*ph*, 101
Grilled Salmon with Sweet Balsamic Onions, 118
Grilled Sirloin Salad, 75

H

Hamburger Sliders with Dijon Mustard Sauce, 9
Herbal Ice Cubes, 60

I

Indian Lamb Curry, 102
Italian Minestrone, 54
Italian Sausage and White Bean Soup, 55

J

Jamaican Chicken Thighs, 103

L

Lemon Garlic Shrimp, 119
Lemon Scones, 159

M

Malaysian Shrimp with Pineapple, 104
Maple Apples, 29
Maple Glazed Pork Loin, 76–77

O

Old Fashioned Peanut Butter Cookies, 162
Orange Glazed Cornish Hens, 78
Oven Fried Cod, 79
Oven Pork Stew with Sweet Potatoes and Shallots, 56, 57*ph*

P

Pan Grilled Beef with Mushroom Gravy, 80
Parmesan Popovers, 30
Pasta Primavera, 130
Pear-Raisin Streusel Crunch Pie, 160–161
Penne with Broccoli Rabe, Prosciutto, and Garlic, 126*ph*, 131
Pepper Crushed Beef Tenderloin with Horseradish Sauce, 81
Plum Clafouti, 163

Polenta Croutons, 24
Potato Crusted Bacon Quiche, 120*ph*, 121
Potato Frittata, 122
Provençal Fish Stew, 106

R

Raspberry Ice Cream Floats, 164
Raspberry Vinegar, 40
Really Quick Pancetta Penne, 132
Red Bean Casserole, 123
Ribollita, 42*ph*, 58
Rigatoni with Sausage, 133
Roast Beef Hash, 82
Roast Beef Reubens, 83
Roast Chicken, 84
Roasted Carrot Soup, 59
Roasted Chickpeas, 10
Roasted Potatoes, Carrots and Parsnips, 31
Rustic Garlic and Olive Oil Mashed Potatoes, 32

S

Saffron Asparagus Risotto with Peas, 33
Salmon Quinoa Risotto, 110*ph*, 124
Sausage Stuffed Mushrooms, 11
Savory Ginger Beef BBQ Appetizer, 14
Shrimp and Pasta Bowl with Feta, 135
Shrimp Martinis, 4
Shrimp Provençal, 125
Slow Cooked BBQ Chicken, 86–87
Spaghetti Agli Olio, 134
Spaghetti Bolognese, 136
Spaghetti Carbonara, 137
Spaghetti Squash with Pine Nuts and Sage, 34*ph*, 35
Spanish Chicken with Red Peppers, 107

Spanish Style Dates with Bacon, 12*ph*, 13
Spiced Beef Stew with Dried Fruits, 85
Spiced Sweet Potato Wedges, 36
Spinach with Golden Raisins, 37
Steamed New Potatoes with Creamy Herb Dressing, 38
Straw and Hay, 138, 139*ph*
Stuffed Shells Florentine, 140
Sweet and Sour Pork, 108
Sweet Onion, White Bean, and Artichoke Dip, 15
Sweet Potato and Squash Mash, 39

T

Tagliatelle with Creamy Goat Cheese Sauce, 141
Tapioca Rice and Rhubarb Pudding, 165
Tarragon Vinegar, 40
Tasty Tortilla Soup, 60
Tomato, Basil and Mozzarella Salad, 40
Traditional Lump Crab Cakes, 88*ph*, 89
Triple Gingerbread Squares, 166*ph*, 167
Tuna Dip, 10
Turkey Pesto Sandwiches, 90
Turkey Stroganoff, 91

V

Vanilla Angel Cake, 168
Vanilla Custard with Blueberry Sauce, 169
Vegetable Provencal Tart, 92*ph*, 109
Veggie Dip, 6
Veggie Pita Triangles, 4
Vinegar, 40

W

Wild Mushroom Soup, 61

Subject Index

NOTE: Page numbers followed by a *ph* refer to photographs. Page ranges in **bold** refer to chapters.

A

alcohol, 150

almonds, 12*ph*, 13, 144, 148, 163

American Classics, **63–91**

  BBQ Beef Sandwiches, 64

  Chicken Joes, 62*ph*, 65

  Chicken Pot Pie with Phyllo, 66–67

  Classic Free-Formed Meatloaf, 68

  Classic Grilled Cheese, 69

  Classic Mac 'n' Cheese, 70–71

  Everyday Taco Salad, 72

  Filet Mignon with Spiced Pepper Crust, 73

  Grilled Lamb Burgers, 74

  Grilled Sirloin Salad, 75

  Maple Glazed Pork Loin, 76–77

  Orange Glazed Cornish Hens, 78

  Oven Fried Cod, 79

  Pan Grilled Beef with Mushroom Gravy, 80

  Pepper Crushed Beef Tenderloin with Horseradish Sauce, 81

  Roast Beef Hash, 82

  Roast Beef Reubens, 83

  Roast Chicken, 84

  Slow Cooked BBQ Chicken, 86–87

  Spiced Beef Stew with Dried Fruits, 85

  Traditional Lump Crab Cakes, 88*ph*, 89

  Turkey Pesto Sandwiches, 90

  Turkey Stroganoff, 91

angel cake, 168

appetizers. See Starters

apple, 18–19, 29, 59, 84, 145, 146*ph*, 147–150

apple juice, 86–87

apricots, dried, 85, 117, 145

Arborio rice, 33

aromatic nut oils, 19

artichoke hearts, 4, 15

Asian flavors, 105

asparagus, 33, 49, 130, 171

B

bacon, 12*ph*, 13, 120*ph*, 121

balsamic vinegar, 118

banana, 39, 149, 151

barbecue sauce, 62*ph*, 64–65, 86–87

basil, 40

basil vinegar, 40

beans

  black, 22, 23*ph*, 47, 116

  canned, 119

  cannellini, 15, 53–55, 58

  chickpeas, 4, 10, 48–49, 97–98

  green, 130, 171

  lima, 25

  red, 123

  white, 15, 53–55, 58

beef

  Baked Potato Soup, 46

  BBQ Beef Sandwiches, 64

  Chinese Five-Spice Steak with Chinese Noodles, 96

  Classic Free-Formed Meatloaf, 68

  Everyday Taco Salad, 72

  Filet Mignon with Spiced Pepper Crust, 73

  Grilled Sirloin Salad, 75

  Pan Grilled Beef with Mushroom Gravy, 80

  Pepper Crushed Beef Tenderloin with Horseradish Sauce, 81

  Roast Beef Hash, 82

  Roast Beef Reubens, 83

  Savory Ginger Beef BBQ Appetizer, 14

  Spaghetti Bolognese, 136

  Spiced Beef Stew with Dried Fruits, 85

beets, 171

biscotti, 144

black beans, 22, 23*ph*, 47, 116

blueberry, 148, 169

bread

  breadcrumbs, 26, 55, 68, 70–71, 79, 81, 89

  buns, 9

  French, 4

  French rolls, 90

  hamburger buns, 62*ph*, 64–65

  Italian, 26

  panko breadcrumbs, 79

  pita, 4, 9, 97

  sourdough, 20

whole-wheat, 69

whole-wheat cocktail buns, 9

breadcrumbs, 26, 55, 68, 70–71, 79, 81, 89

broccoli, 50*ph*, 51, 120*ph*, 121, 126*ph*, 171

broccoli rabe, 131

brownies, 156–157

brussel sprouts, 171

buns, 9

butternut squash, 39, 48

C

cabbage, 19, 54, 58, 171

cake, 168

cannellini beans, 15, 53–55, 58

cannelloni, 140

canola oil, 19

capelli d'angelo, 140

carrots, 27, 31, 59, 171

cashews, 44

cauliflower, 26, 58, 102, 172

celery, 172

cheddar cheese, 3, 46, 50*ph*, 51, 60, 69–71

cheese
cheddar, 3, 46, 50*ph*, 51, 60, 69–71
cooking with, viii, 69
cream, 6, 10, 142*ph*, 154–155
feta, 28, 74, 135
fontina, 8
goat, 141
gorgonzola, 18
low-fat, 4
mascarpone, 24

Mexican, 100*ph*, 101
mozzarella, 40
parmesan, 24–26, 30, 32, 52, 54
ricotta, 137, 140–141

cheesecake, 142*ph*, 154–155

cherries, 114, 152, 153*ph*, 164

chicken
Asian Chicken Dumplings, 2
Asopao De Pollo— Puerto Rican Chicken and Rice Soup, 45
Caesar Salad with Chicken, 20
Caramelized Onion Chicken, 113
Chicken and Noodle Salad with Peanut Dressing, 129
Chicken Cacciatore, 94
Chicken Joes, 62*ph*, 65
Chicken Paprikash, 95
Chicken Pot Pie with Phyllo, 66–67
Chicken with White Wine Garlic Sauce, 115
Country Captain Chicken, 117
Jamaican Chicken Thighs, 103
Red Bean Casserole, 123
Roast Chicken, 84
Slow Cooked BBQ Chicken, 86–87
Spanish Chicken with Red Peppers, 107

chicken livers, 136

chickpeas, 4, 10, 48–49, 97–98

Chinese five-spice powder, 96

Chinese noodles, 96

chives, 52

chocolate, 145, 150–152, 153*ph*, 156–158, 164

chutney, 10

cilantro, 22, 23*ph*, 74

cinnamon, 36

clafouti, 163

clams, 10

club soda, 164

cocoa, 156–157

coconut, 145

cod, 79

Comfort Food Starters. *See* Starters

conchiglie, 140

cook time, 87

cookies, 162

cooking oil, 19

cooking tips, 87

Cornish hens, 78

cottage cheese, 142*ph*, 154–155

crab, 5–6, 88*ph*, 89

crab cakes, 88*ph*, 89

cranberries, 59, 145, 159

cream cheese, 6, 10, 142*ph*, 154–155

cremini mushrooms, 11

crookneck squash, 173

croutons, 20, 24, 55

crust, 161

curry, 6, 102, 116

custard, 169

D

dates, 12*ph*, 13
Desserts, **143–167**
  Almond Biscotti, 144
  Ambrosia, 145
  Apple Blueberry
    Almond Crisp, 148
  Apple Pandowdy,
    146*ph*, 147
  Baked Apples with Figs,
    149
  Banana Chocolate Chip
    Muffins, 151
  Chocolate Cherry
    Pudding, 152, 153*ph*
  Chunky Applesauce,
    150
  Classic Cheesecake,
    142*ph*, 154–155
  Double Chocolate
    Brownies, 156–157
  Fudge Pudding, 158
  Lemon Scones, 159
  Old Fashioned Peanut
    Butter Cookies, 162
  Pear-Raisin Streusel
    Crunch Pie, 160–161
  Plum Clafouti, 163
  Raspberry Ice Cream
    Floats, 164
  Tapioca Rice and
    Rhubarb Pudding, 165
  Triple Gingerbread
    Squares, 166*ph*, 167
  Vanilla Angel Cake, 168
  Vanilla Custard with
    Blueberry Sauce, 169
dijon mustard, x *ph*, 7, 9
dill, 6
dips, 6, 10
dittali, 140

dressing, 38, 40
dried fruits, 85

E

eggplant, 21
eggs, 7, 122
English cucumber, 28
entrées. *See* American
  Classics; International;
  One Pot; Pasta; Skillet
escarole, 53
extra virgin olive oil, 19

F

falafel, 97
farfalle, 140
fat, viii, 19, 44
fennel, 25, 59
feta cheese, 28, 74, 135
fettuccine, 138, 139*ph*,
  140
figs, 149, 164
filet mignon, 73
fish, 79, 106, 118–119
5-Minute Creamy
  Mushroom Soup, 44
five-spice powder, 96
French bread, 4
French rolls, 90
fruit puree, 155
fusilli, 135, 140

G

garbanzo beans. *See*
  chickpeas
garlic, 32, 87, 98, 115,
  119, 126*ph*, 131
garlic vinegar, 40
gemelli, 141
ginger, 14, 27, 105, 150,
  166*ph*, 167

gingersnap, 164
gnocchi, 98, 141
goat cheese, 141
golden raisins, 27, 37
gorgonzola cheese, 18
grains, 119
Greek yogurt, 4, 6, 47, 52,
  97, 142*ph*, 154–155,
  164
green beans, 130, 171
greens, 37, 75, 172
grilled cheese, 69

H

half-and-half, 52, 61
ham, 137–138, 139*ph*
hamburger, 174 *ph*, 9
hamburger buns, 62*ph*,
  64–65
hash; 82
hash browns, 120*ph*,
  121
herbs, 25, 38, 52, 60, 113,
  150
horseradish, 81
hummus, 4

I

ice cream, 164
ice cubes, 60
International, **93–109**
  Chicken Cacciatore, 94
  Chicken Paprikash, 95
  Chinese Five-Spice
    Steak with Chinese
    Noodles, 96
  Falafel, 97
  Gnocchi with
    Tomatoes, Chickpeas,
    and Spinach, 98
  Greek Lamb Chops, 99

Grilled Pork and Cheese Quesadillas, 100*ph*, 101
Indian Lamb Curry, 102
Jamaican Chicken Thighs, 103
Malaysian Shrimp with Pineapple, 104
Provencal Fish Stew, 106
Spanish Chicken with Red Peppers, 107
Sweet and Sour Pork, 108
Vegetable Provencal Tart, 92*ph*, 109
Italian sausage, 55, 128, 133

J

Jerusalem artichokes, 25
jicama, 25

K

kalamata olives, 28
kohlrabi, 172

L

lamb, 34*ph*, 74, 99, 102
lasagne, 141
lemon, 27, 119, 159
lentils, 119
lima beans, 25
lime, 22, 23*ph*
linguine, 129, 141
lumache, 141

M

macaroni, 141
mac 'n' cheese, 70–71

main courses. *See* American Classics; International; One Pot; Pasta; Skillet
maple syrup, 29, 76–77
marinara sauce, 128, 132, 140
marmalade, 78
marshmallow, 145
mascarpone cheese, 24
meatballs, 112
meatloaf, 68
Mexican cheese, 100*ph*, 101
molasses, 166*ph*, 167
mozzarella cheese, 40
muffins, 151
mushrooms, 11, 44, 61, 80, 172

N

nut oils, 19
nuts, 34*ph*, 35, 37, 44

O

oil, 19
olive oil, 19, 32
olives, 28
One Pot, **111–125**
Baked Turkey Meatballs, 112
with beans, 125
Country Captain Chicken, 117
with grains, 125
Grilled Salmon with Sweet Balsamic Onions, 118
Red Bean Casserole, 123
with rice, 125

Salmon Quinoa Risotto, 124
onion
Caramelized Onion Chicken, 113
cooking with, 87
Grilled Salmon with Sweet Balsamic Onions, 118
red, 6
selecting and storing, 172
sweet, 15
orange, 78, 145
orecchiette, 141
oregano, 99
orzo, 49
oyster sauce, 14

P

pancetta bacon, 132
pans, 87
papparadelle, 141
paprika, 95
parmesan cheese, 24–26, 30, 32, 54
parsley, 87
parsnips, 31, 172
pasta, 54, 70–71, 87, 91, 95–96, 115, 140
Pasta, **127–141**
Baked Ziti, 128
Chicken and Noodle Salad with Peanut Dressing, 129
Pasta Primavera, 130
Penne with Broccoli Rabe, Prosciutto, and Garlic, 126*ph*, 131
Really Quick Pancetta Penne, 132

Rigatoni with Sausage, 133

Shrimp and Pasta Bowl with Feta, 135

Spaghetti Agli Olio, 134

Spaghetti Bolognese, 136

Spaghetti Carbonara, 137

Straw and Hay, 138, 139*ph*

Stuffed Shells Florentine, 140

Tagliatelle with Creamy Goat Cheese Sauce, 141

pastry dough, 161

peanut butter, 48, 129, 162

peanut oil, 19

pear, 160–161

peas, 33, 130, 138, 139*ph*, 170*ph*

penne, 130–132, 135, 141

pepper

  bell, 172

  black, 81

  cracked black, 73

  green, 62*ph*, 65

  red, 6, 25, 107

  yellow, 25, 28

pesto sauce, 90

phyllo, 66–67

pie, 160–161

pine nuts, 34*ph*, 35, 37

pineapple, 104, 108

pita bread, 4, 9, 97

pizza, 8

plums, 163

polenta, 24

popcorn, 52

popovers, 30

pork, 56, 57*ph*, 68, 76–77, 100*ph*, 101, 108, 114

pot pie, 66–67

potatoes

  Baked Potato Soup, 46

  Cheddar Baked Potato Skins, 3

  Potato Crusted Bacon Quiche, 120*ph*, 121

  Potato Frittata, 122

  Roast Beef Hash, 82

  Roasted Potatoes, Carrots, and Parsnips, 31

  Rustic Garlic and Olive Oil Mashed Potatoes, 32

  selecting and storing, 173

  Steamed New Potatoes with Creamy Herb Dressing, 38

poultry. *See under individual type*

pretzels, 52

prosciutto, 54, 126*ph*, 131

prunes, dried, 85

pudding, 152, 153*ph*, 158, 165, 169

Q

quinoa, 124

R

raisins, 27, 37, 160–161

raspberry vinegar, 40

raspberries, 163–164

red bean, 123

Reuben, 83

rhubarb, 165

ribollita, 42

rice, 33, 45, 116–117, 125, 165

ricotta cheese, 137, 140–141, 145

rigatoni, 133, 141

risotto, 33, 124

roast beef, 82–83

roast chicken, 84

Rock Cornish hens, 78

S

saffron, 33

sage, 34*ph*, 35

Salad, **17–40**

  Apple and Gorgonzola Cheese Salad, 18

  Caesar Salad with Chicken, 20

  Chicken and Noodle Salad with Peanut Dressing, 129

  Chopped Salad with Cilantro Lime Dressing, 22, 23*ph*

  Everyday Taco Salad, 72

  Greek Country Salad, 28

  Grilled Sirloin Salad, 75

  Tomato, Basil & Mozzarella Salad, 40

salmon, 118, 124

salt, viii–ix, 150

sandwiches, 64, 69, 83, 90

sauces, 119, 132

sauerkraut, 83

sausage, 11, 55, 128, 133
sauté, 77
scallions, 105, 173
scones, 159
seafood, 88*ph*, 89, 104, 106, 119, 125, 135
serrano ham, 137
sesame oil, 19
sesame tahini, 4
shallots, 56, 57*ph*, 173
shrimp, 4, 104, 106, 119, 125, 135
Sides, **17–40**
  Braised Cabbage and Apples, 19
  Classic Ratatouille, 16*ph*, 21
  Costa Rican Black Beans and Rice (Gallo Pinto), 116
  Creamy Polenta, 24
  Creamy Succotash, 25
  Crispy Roasted Cauliflower, 26
  Ginger Carrots with Golden Raisins and Lemon, 27
  Maple Apples, 29
  Parmesan Popovers, 30
  Roasted Potatoes, Carrots, and Parsnips, 31
  Rustic Garlic and Olive Oil Mashed Potatoes, 32
  Saffron Asparagus Risotto with Peas, 33
  Spaghetti Squash with Pine Nuts and Sage, 35

Spiced Sweet Potato Wedges, 36
Spinach with Golden Raisins, 37
Steamed New Potatoes with Creamy Herb Dressing, 38
Sweet Potato and Squash Mash, 39
Skillet, **111–125**
  Caramelized Onion Chicken, 113
  Cherry Glazed Pork Loin Chops, 114
  Chicken with White Wine Garlic Sauce, 115
  Costa Rican Black Beans and Rice (Gallo Pinto), 116
  Lemon Garlic Shrimp, 119
  Potato Crusted Bacon Quiche, 120*ph*, 121
  Potato Frittata, 122
  Salmon Quinoa Risotto, 110*ph*
  Shrimp Provençal, 125
soba noodles, 129
sodium, viii–ix
Soups, **43–61**
  Asopao De Pollo—Puerto Rican Chicken and Rice Soup, 45
  Baked Potato Soup, 46
  Black Bean Soup with a Kick, 47
  Cheddar Cheese and Broccoli Soup, 50*ph*, 51

  Chickpea Soup with Orzo, 49
  Creamy Tomato Soup, 52
  Escarole and White Bean Soup, 53
  fat, skimming, 44
  5-Minute Creamy Mushroom Soup, 44
  flavor test, 51
  freezing, 46
  Italian Minestrone, 54
  Italian Sausage and White Bean Soup, 55
  Ribollita, 58
  Roasted Carrot Soup, 59
  Tasty Tortilla Soup, 60
  toppings, 52
  Wild Mushroom Soup, 61
sour cream, 7
sourdough bread, 20
soy sauce, 105
spaghetti, 134, 136–137, 141
spaghetti squash, 34*ph*, 35
spices, 87, 103, 113, 150
spinach, 37, 98, 134, 140
Splenda, ix
squash, 35, 39, 48, 60, 173
Starters, **1–15**
  Asian Chicken Dumplings, 2
  Cheddar Baked Potato Skins, 3
  Cheese and Fruit Bruschetta, 4

Chutney Dip, 10
Clam Dip, 10
Classic Hummus, 4
Crab Louis, 5
Creamy Crab Spread, 6
Creamy Deviled Eggs, 7
Curry Dip, 6
Dill Dip, 6
Double Cheese Pizza Bites, 8
Hamburger Sliders with Dijon Mustard Sauce, 9
Roasted Chickpeas, 10
Sausage Stuffed Mushrooms, 11
Savory Ginger Beef BBQ Appetizer, 14
Shrimp Martinis, 4
Spanish Style Dates with Bacon, 12*ph*, 13
Sweet Onion, White Bean, and Artichoke Dip, 15
Tuna Dip, 10
Veggie Dip, 6
Veggie Pita Triangles, 4
steak, 46, 64
stevia, ix
Stews, **43–61**
   Butternut Squash Stew with Chickpeas, 48
   flavor test, 51

freezing, 46
Oven Pork Stew with Sweet Potatoes and Shallots, 56, 57*ph*
Provençal Fish Stew, 106
Spiced Beef Stew with Dried Fruits, 85
   toppings, 52
stocking up, 119
streusel, 160–161
stroganoff, 91
succotash, 25
sugar, ix
summer squash, 173
sun-dried tomatoes, 25, 33, 131
sweet and sour pork, 108
sweet potatoes, 36, 39, 56, 57*ph*
sweetener, ix

T

taco salad, 72
tagliatelle pasta, 141
tapioca, 165
tarragon vinegar, 40
tart, 92*ph*, 109
tomatoes, 40, 52, 62*ph*, 65, 92*ph*, 109, 119, 173
tomatoes, sun-dried, 25, 33, 131
tortilla chips, 72

tortillas, 60, 100*ph*, 101
tuna, 10
turkey, 90–91, 112
turkey sausage, 55
turnips, 173

U

udon noodles, 129

V

vanilla, 150, 168–169
veal, 68
vegetables, 171
vermicelli, 141
vinegar, 40, 87

W

white beans, 15, 53–55, 58
wine, 115, 125
wonton wrappers, 2

Y

yeast, 8
yellow squash, 173
yogurt, 4, 6, 47, 52, 97, 142*ph*, 154–155, 164

Z

ziti, 128
zucchini, 21, 54, 62*ph*, 65, 92*ph*, 109, 173